Essentials of Oral Histology and Embryology

A Clinical Approach

RK 280 .A84 1992

Avery, James K.

Essentials of oral histology
  and embryology

D0207263

Essentials of Oral Histology and Embryology
A Clinical Approach

JAMES K. AVERY, D.D.S., Ph.D.

Professor of Dentistry, School of Dentistry;
Professor of Anatomy, Medical School
University of Michigan
Ann Arbor, Michigan

Edited by

PAULINE F. STEELE, B.S., R.D.H., B.S. (Educ.), M.A.

Director and Professor Emeritus—Dental Hygiene
University of Michigan, School of Dentistry
Ann Arbor, Michigan

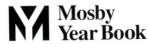 **Mosby Year Book**

St. Louis Baltimore Boston Chicago London Philadelphia Sydney Toronto

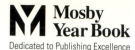

Mosby
Year Book
Dedicated to Publishing Excellence

Editor: Robert Reinhardt
Project Manager: Barbara Merritt
Cover Design: Gail Morey Hudson

Copyright © 1992 by Mosby–Year Book, Inc.
A Mosby imprint of Mosby–Year Book, Inc.

All rights reserved. No part of this publication may be reproduced, stored in a retrieval system, or transmitted, in any form or by any means, electronic, mechanical, photocopying, recording, or otherwise, without prior written permission from the publisher.

Permission to photocopy or reproduce solely for internal or personal use is permitted for libraries or other users registered with the Copyright Clearance Center, provided that the base fee of $4.00 per chapter plus $.10 per page is paid directly to the Copyright Clearance Center, 27 Congress Street, Salem, MA 01970. This consent does not extend to other kinds of copying, such as copying for general distribution, for advertising or promotional purposes, for creating new collected works, or for resale.

Printed in the United States of America

Mosby–Year Book, Inc.
11830 Westline Industrial Drive
St. Louis, MO 63146

International Standard Book Number: 0-8016-5868

95 96 CG/CD/WA 9 8 7 6 5 4

Acknowledgments

Numerous colleagues have provided valuable contributions in preparation of this textbook, *Essentials of Oral Histology and Embryology: A Clinical Approach*. I am indebted for their assistance and wish to acknowledge with gratitude each of these authors for their permission to use materials. Individual colleague contributions have been personally recognized in the respective chapter where it appears.

Through the interest and encouragement of colleagues and students at the University of Michigan, the concept of visual and didactic material being placed in proximity was initiated. Organizationally, a concerted effort was made to produce a book for the dental professional that includes fundamental theories of microscopic anatomy for this subject area.

I am most appreciative for the excellent artwork contributed to the book by Alayne Evans and Chris Jung, Medical Illustrators, at the School of Dentistry, University of Michigan. This book has been enhanced through Dr. Donald S. Strachan's expertise in scientific data presentation and analysis. I extend my sincere thanks to all who assisted with the publication. It is hoped that these efforts will provide worthwhile experiences for teachers, students, and practitioners using this text.

James K. Avery

Preface

This textbook's purpose is to familiarize dental professionals with knowledge in the fields of oral histology and embryology pertinent to clinical dental hygiene and dental practice. Developmental and structural microscopic anatomy are significant sciences for the practitioner. In acquiring an understanding of how cells, tissues, and organs develop and function, one gains a clearer perspective of these structures and for the basis of their treatment.

Oral histology and embryology are most relevant sciences to the understanding of clinical oral manifestations. Therefore the text has been designed to encompass histologic and embryologic information with specific consideration of clinical connotations. This textbook has been written especially for dental hygiene students, practitioners, educators, and other co-associated professionals.

Several special features are found in this text. Numerous color photographs enhance visual learning. A concerted effort has been made to place all illustrative material as close as possible to the explanatory text. Each chapter has an overview to give a perspective of the chapter content, followed by more detailed descriptions of basic principles of oral histology and embryology and their relationships to clinical practice. This emphasis enables formation of both a practical and a theoretical approach to these essential sciences. Diagrams throughout the text facilitate further comprehension. Also included are low magnification light and high magnification electron microscopic photographs to assist with learning and clarify concepts. A glossary has been included to agument learning.

Professional competence connotes more than technical ability. Therefore an effort has been made to indicate those aspects of basic sciences that complement the technical procedures. Dental professionals must understand and appreciate these concepts involving clinical practice.

Pauline F. Steele

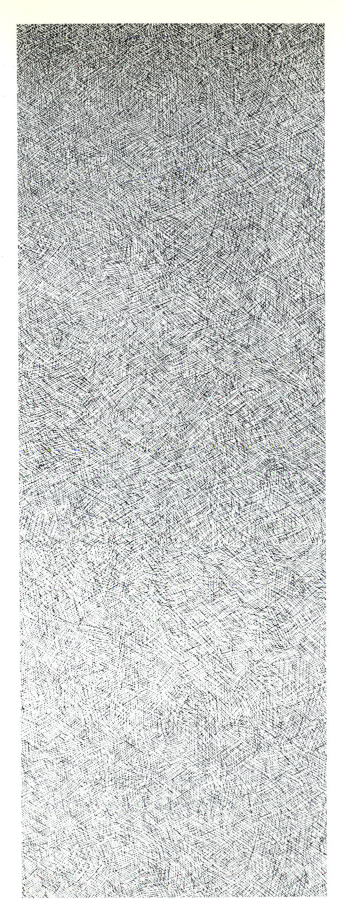

Contents

Essentials of Oral Histology and Embryology

A Clinical Approach

Development and Structure of Cells and Tissues

■ Overview

The smallest unit of structure is the cell, composed of a nucleus and cytoplasm. The nucleus contains the nucleic acids DNA and RNA, the fundamental structures of life. The cytoplasm functions in absorption and cell duplication, in which numerous organelles in the cytoplasm perform specific actions. The cell cycle is the time required for the DNA to duplicate before mitosis. This chapter discusses the four stages of mitosis—prophase, metaphase, anaphase, and telophase. Next, the three periods of prenatal development—proliferative, embryonic, and fetal—are described. The fertilization of the ovum and its implantation in the uterine wall are discussed. In addition, the origin of the human tissues—ectoderm, mesoderm, and endoderm—is presented, followed by the differentiation of tissue types, such as epithelium and skin with its derivatives, and the central and peripheral nervous systems. Finally, the development of connective tissues of the body such as fibrous tissue, cartilage, bone, muscles, and the cardiovascular system is delineated. After reading this chapter, one should better comprehend the origin, development, and organization of the various cells and tissues of the human body.

1

■ *Cell Structure and Function*

The human body is composed of cells, intercellular substance, or the products of these cells, and fluid that bathes tissues. Cells are the smallest living units capable of independent existence. They carry out functions of the vital processes of **absorption, assimilation, respiration, irritability, conductivity, growth, reproduction,** and **excretion.** Cells vary in size, shape, and structure, and these components relate to cell function. Regardless of function, each cell has a number of characteristics in common with other cells such as the nucleus and the cytoplasm. Cells are composed of a **nucleus,** containing a **nucleolus,** and the **cytoplasm,** which surrounds the nucleus. The shape of a cell may be related to its function. A cell on the surface of the skin, for example, serves best as a thin, flattened disc, whereas a respiratory cell is cuboidal or columnar to facilitate adsorption, with mobile cilia to move fluid from the lung to the oropharynx. Surrounding each cell is the **intercellular** material that provides the cell with nutrition and takes up waste products; it also provides the body with form. It may be as soft as loose connective tissue or as hard as bone cartilage or teeth. **Fluid,** the third component of the body, is the blood and lymph that travel throughout the body in vessels or the tissue fluid that bathes each cell and fiber of the body.

Cell Nucleus

A nucleus is found in all cells except mature red blood cells and blood platelets. The nucleus is usually round to ovoid, depending on the cell's shape. Ordinarily, a cell has a single nucleus; however, it may be binucleate, as are cardiac muscle and parenchymal liver cells, or multinucleate, as are osteoclasts and skeletal muscle cells. The nucleus contains nucleic acids, the basis of life, and is important in the production of **deoxyribonucleic acid (DNA)** and **ribonucleic acid (RNA).** DNA contains the genetic information in the cell, and RNA carries this information from the DNA to the sites of actual protein synthesis, which are located in the cell cytoplasm. The nucleus is bound by a membrane, the **nuclear envelope,** which has an opening at the nuclear pore. This envelope is associated with the endoplasmic reticulum of the surrounding cytoplasm, which forms at the end of each cell division. The nucleus contains from one to four nucleoli, which are round, dense bodies constituting the RNA contained in the nucleus. It has no limiting membrane (Figure 1.1).

Cell Cytoplasm

Cytoplasm contains structures necessary for the process of adsorption and production of the cell products. The cytoplasm contains **endoplasmic reticulum (ER),** a system of parallel membrane-bound cavities in the cytoplasm that contain newly acquired and synthesized protein. There are two types of ER: smooth-surfaced and granular or rough-surfaced. Smooth and granular ER can be found in the same cell. The rough surface is caused by the location of ribosomes on the surface of the reticulum and is the site protein production is initiated. Proteins are vital to the cell's metabolic processes, and each type of protein is made up of a number and variety of amino acids linked in a specific sequence. Amino acids form protein-containing groups, which in turn form acids or bases.

Ribosomes are particles that translate genetic codes for proteins and activate mechanisms for their production. They can be found free in the cytoplasm, clustered as polyribosomes, or attached to the ER membranes. Ribosomes are nonspecific as to what type of protein they synthesize. This specificity is dependent on messenger RNA (mRNA), which carries the message directly from DNA of the nucleus to the RNA of the ER. This molecule attaches to the ribosomes and gives orders on the formation of specific amino acids.

The ER transports substances in the cell. Then the ER is connected to the Golgi's apparatus via small vesicles. The **Golgi's apparatus** or **complex** functions in sorting, condensing, packaging, and delivering proteins arriving from the ER. The Golgi's apparatus is composed of cisternae (flat plates), or saccules; small vesicles; and large vacuoles. From here the secretory vesicles move or flow to the cell surface, where they fuse with the cell membrane, the plasmalemma, and release their contents by exocytosis.

Lysosomes are small membrane-bound bodies that contain a variety of acid hydrolase and digestive enzymes that function in breaking down substances both inside and outside the cell. They are in all cells except red blood cells but are prominent in macrophages and leukocytes.

Mitochondria are membrane-bound organelles that lie free in the cytoplasm and are present in all cells. They are important in generating energy and are a major source of adenosine triphosphate (ATP), and therefore the site of many metabolic reactions. These organelles appear as spheres, rods, ovoids, or threadlike bodies. Usually, the inner layer of their trilaminar bounding membrane inflects to form transverse-appearing plates, the cristae (Figure 1.1). Mitochondria lie adjacent to the area that requires their energy production.

Microtubules are small tubular structures in the cytoplasm and are composed of the protein tubulin. These structures may appear singular, as doublets, or as triplets. They likely have function as structural and force-generating elements, and they relate to cilia (motile cell processes) and to centrioles in relation to mitosis. They have cytoskeletal functions in maintaining cell shape. **Centrioles** are short cylinders appearing near the nucleus. Their walls are composed of nine triplets, sets of three microtubules. Centrioles are microtubule-generating centers and are important in mitosis, self-replicating before mitosis begins.

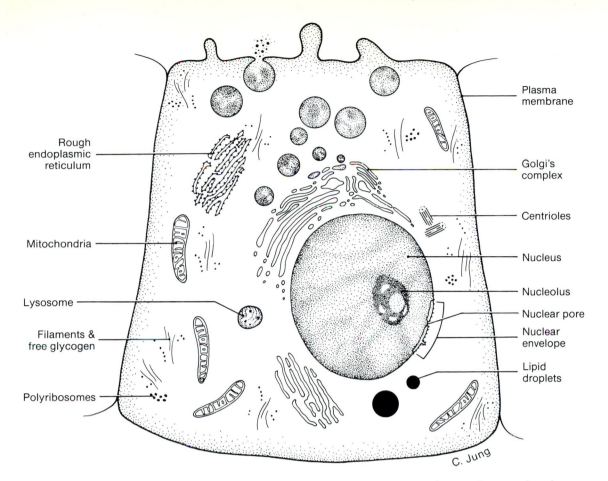

C. Jung

Figure 1.1 *Schematic diagram of cell structure illustrating components such as nucleus, rough endo-plasmic reticulum, mitochondria, Golgi's complex, and centrioles as viewed by electron microscopy.*

Surrounding the cell is the **plasma membrane,** plas-malemma, which envelops the cell and provides a selective barrier that regulates transport of substances into and out of the cell. All membranes are composed mainly of lipid and protein with a small amount of carbohydrate. The plasma membrane also receives signals from hormones and neu-rotransmitters. In addition, cells contain proteins, lipids, or fatty substances that provide energy in the cell and are important components of cell membranes and per-meability. Carbohydrates are also important in cells as the most available energy reserve in the body. They may exist as polysaccharides, polysaccharide-protein complexes, glycoproteins, and glycolipids. These compounds are im-portant in cell function as well as in development of cell products such as supportive tissues and body lubricants.

■ *Cell Division*

Cell Cycle

Cell division is a continuous series of discrete steps by which the cell component divides. This function is related to the need for growth or replacement of tissues and is in part dependent on the length of the cells' life. Cells that are continually renewing are those lining the gastrointestinal tract, those composing the epidermis, and those of the bone marrow. A second type of cell is part of an expanding population—the cells of the kidney, liver, and some glands. The third type of cell does not undergo cell division or, therefore, DNA synthesis—for example, neurons of the adult nervous system. For a somatic cell to undergo cell division, it must pass through a **cell cycle,** which ensures a period of time for DNA genetic material in the daughter cells to duplicate that of its parent cell. However, in a sex cell, ovum or spermatozoon, the process of **meiosis** takes place in which there is a reduction division of the chromosomes in the daughter cell. The result is half as many chromosomes in the daughter cells as in the parent cell. Through this process, after fertilization of the ova by the male chromosomes, the original (diploid) number of chromosomes will be regained. The duration of the cell cycle in somatic cells is known today (Figure 1.2). After mitosis, the cells enter the preduplication or **G1 stage** of the interphase, resting stage, which is the initial stage. This is followed by the **S phase,** where DNA synthesis is completed. Next, the cell enters the **G2 stage** or quiescent phase of post-DNA duplication, and this proceeds into the mitotic stages of prophase, metaphase, anaphase, and telophase (Figure 1.3). The cells then re-enter and remain in the interphase stage until duplication resumes the mitotic process of developing two daughter cells identical to the parent cells.

Mitosis

Before mitosis the cell exists in the interphase as seen in Figure 1.3*A.* The first step of mitosis is **prophase,** in which four changes in structure occur (Figure 1.3*B*). The chromatin thread of the nucleus becomes thickened into rodlike structures called **chromosomes.** Each chromosome then splits in half, and the halves are known as **chromatids.** These line up along the central area of the cell, called the **equatorial plate.** Each chromatid pair is attached to a spherical body termed a **centromere.** As the centriole pair duplicates, there is migration to opposite ends of the cell, accompanied by the chromatids. Those fibers not formed between the migrating centrioles are termed **spindle fibers,** and those that form around each pair of centrioles are termed **astral rays** or **asters** (Figure 1.3*C*). At this time, the nucleolus disappears, and its components become attached to the chromatids. Finally, the nuclear envelope breaks down, changing into granular elements like the endoplasmic reticulum (Figure 1.3*D*).

Upon reaching the **metaphase** stage, the chromatids have moved to the cell center and become arranged along an equatorial plate at right angles to the long axis of the spindle (Figure 1.3*E*). The two chromatids of each chromosome become attached centrally at the equatorial plate to a centromere, with their arms sticking outward. These chromatids then split at the centromere into two sets of chromosomes.

In **anaphase,** the daughter chromosomes move to the opposite poles of the cell, with the full complement of 46 at each end (Figure 1.3*F* and *G*). This is thought to occur by movement of the chromosomal microtubules that attract

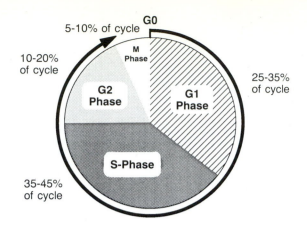

Figure 1.2   *Periods of cell cycle indicate relative amounts of time needed for each phase. G1 is the preduplication, or resting, phase, which takes about 8 to 10 hours. In the S phase, DNA duplication takes place in 6 to 8 hours. The G2 phase is the postduplication phase, which takes about 4 to 6 hours. In the M phase, mitosis occurs, taking 30 to 45 minutes. These figures are for cultured mammalian cells. The total is 18 to 24 hours for the four stages of cytokinesis.*

the chromatids toward the poles. A constriction begins to appear around the midbody of the cell (Figure 1.3*G*).

In **telophase,** the chromosomes detach from the chromosomal microtubules, and the microtubules disintegrate (Figure 1.3*H*). The chromosomes next elongate and disperse, losing their identity and regaining the chromatin thread appearance. Both the nucleoli within the nucleus and the nuclear envelope then reappear. As each nucleus matures, the cleavage furrow deepens in the midcell until the two daughter cells separate (Figure 1.3*H*).

■ *Clinical Comment*

All cells have a limited lifetime. For example, the life span of white blood cells is only a few hours to a few days. However, the red blood cells live approximately 120 days and then are ingested by macrophages. Surface covering cells, such as those of the skin, hair, or nails, renew as they are replaced, as do cells lining the respiratory, urinary, and gastrointestinal tracts. Other cells in the body do not normally renew after maturity unless they are injured, such as the cells of the liver, kidneys, and thyroid gland.

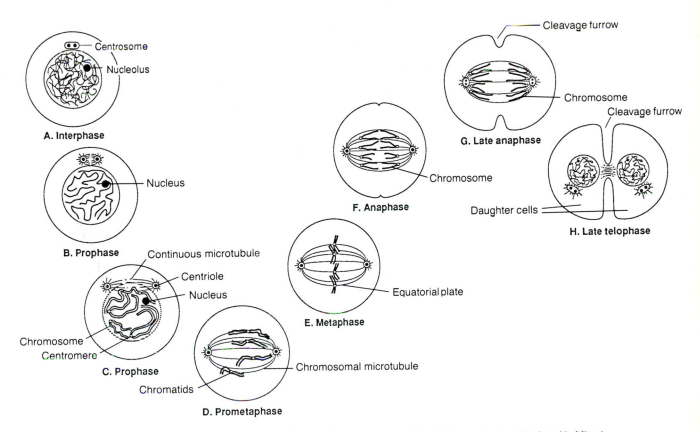

Figure 1.3 *Mitosis of somatic cell. The continuous process of cell division is shown in A to H. Mitosis is replication of parent chromosomes and distribution of two sets of chromosomes into two separate and equal nuclei. The stages are as follows: (A) Interphase, the resting cell. (B and C) During prophase, the chromatin thread shortens, thickens, and becomes chromosomes, which then split into pairs or chromatids. The nuclear membrane disappears, and the centrioles appear and begin migration to the opposite poles of the cell. (D) In the prometaphase, or early metaphase, the chromatid pairs attach to centromere and line up in the equatorial plate of the cell. (E) Metaphase occurs when the centromeres and chromatids line up in middle of cell. Centrioles are at opposite ends of cell and attach to chromosomes by mitotic spindles. (F) Anaphase is a division of centromeres and movement of the completed identical sets of chromatids (chromosomes) to opposite ends of the cells. (G) In late anaphase, identical sets of chromosomes have reached the opposite pole and cell cleavage begins. (H) In telophase, a nuclear membrane reappears, nucleoli appear, and chromosomes lengthen and form a chromatin thread. Mitotic spindles disappear, and centrioles duplicate so that each cell has completely identical properties.*

Proliferative period
0 to 2 weeks

Embryonic period
2 to 8 weeks

Fetal period
8 weeks to 9 months

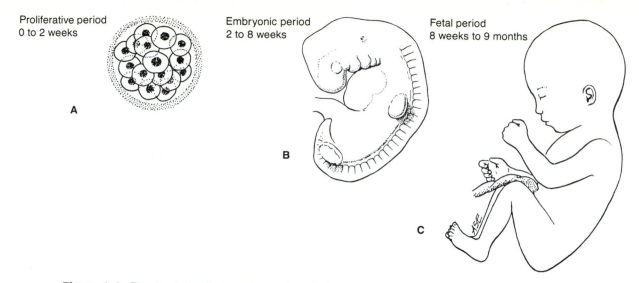

A

B

C

Figure 1.4 *The developing human passes through three periods:* **A,** *The proliferative two-week period, when cell division is prevalent;* **B,** *the embryonic period, which extends from the second to the eighth weeks, and* **C,** *the fetal period from the eighth week to birth.*

■ Origin of Human Tissue

Periods of Prenatal Development

Implantation and enlargement of the blastocyst, which contains the embryonic tissues, occur rapidly and are termed the **proliferative period.** This period persists for the first two weeks. During this time, fertilization, implantation, and formation of the embryonic disc takes place. After the second week, this mass of cells begins to take the form of an embryo, so the period of two to eight weeks is appropriately termed the **embryonic period.** During this period, the different types of tissues develop, organizing to form organ systems located in various areas of the embryo. The heart forms and begins to beat. The face and oral structures develop. At eight weeks, the embryo takes on a more human appearance and passes into the **fetal period,** which extends until birth (Figure 1.4). The increase in body weight and size reflects the beginning of various organs and systems.

Ovarian Cycle, Fertilization, Implantation, and Development of the Embryonic Disc

The origin of tissues begins with fertilization of the egg, or ovum, which occurs when sperm contact the egg in the distal part of the uterine tube (Figure 1.5). The fertilized egg grows and is termed the **zygote.** The cell mass produces a ball of cells, the **morula,** in the uterine tube. The morula begins migration medially to the uterus, reaching it at the end of the first week. The uterine cavity meanwhile was preparing for the arrival of the fertilized ovum by a thickening of the uterine lining, or **endometrium,** and the development of capillaries and glands to nourish the ovum. This cyclical event is under the control of the hormones estrogen and progesterone (Figure 1.6). The morula increases in size and is termed a **blastocyst.** As it swells, it becomes hollow and develops a small inner cell mass. When this ball of cells reaches the uterine cavity, it attaches to the sticky wall and becomes embedded as the surface cells of the zygote digest the endometrium, permitting deeper penetration. This process is known as **implantation** (Figures 1.5 to 1.7).

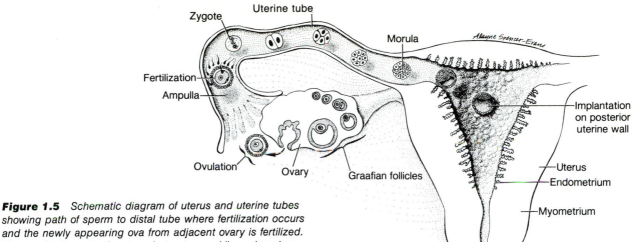

Figure 1.5 *Schematic diagram of uterus and uterine tubes showing path of sperm to distal tube where fertilization occurs and the newly appearing ova from adjacent ovary is fertilized. The resultant zygote then travels to uterus while undergoing cleavage and implantation on seventh day after conception.*

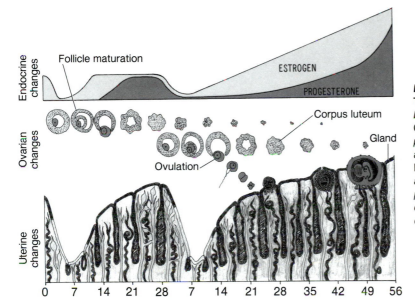

Figure 1.6 *Cyclical events of ovulatory cycle. Top, Endocrine changes: ovulation is controlled by the endocrines estrogen and progesterone. Center, Ovarian changes with maturation and expulsion of ova from ovary on the fourteenth day and implantation in uterine wall seven days later. Bottom, Uterine changes: uterine wall thickens and prepares for implantation each month. If implantation does not occur, the uterine wall erodes with loss of the blood vessels and gland ducts (menstruation).*

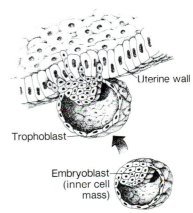

Figure 1.7 *Implantation of fertilized ovum (zygote) in wall of uterus. Outer cells of trophoblast digest uterine cells in order to implant. Embryoblast develops within cell mass and, as cell mass expands, forms a surrounding cavity.*

Two small cavities develop on either side of the inner cell mass, and where they contact in the center, a small disc is formed, termed the **embryonic disc** (Figure 1.8). The embryonic disc becomes the embryo, composed of the common walls of the two adjacent sacs. One sac is lined with **ectodermal** cells, which will form the future outer body covering, or **epithelium.** The other sac is lined with **endodermal** cells. On the dorsal surface of the embryonic disc, the ectoderm gives rise to the **neural plate,** whose lateral boundaries elevate to form a **neural tube** that will form the future brain and spinal cord (Figure 1.9). The endodermal tissue also forms a tube giving rise to the gastrointestinal tract. As this tube elongates, it develops outpouchings forming the pharyngeal pouches of the lung buds, liver, gallbladder, pancreas, and urinary bladder (Figure 1.10A and B).

Next, cells develop between the ectodermal and endodermal layers in the embryonic disc. This area becomes the **mesodermal cell layer.** These cells will develop into the muscles, skeleton, and blood cells of the developing embryo (Figure 1.11). Mesodermal cells also accompany the elongating digestive tube and support its walls with muscle growth. This enables function and aids in the development of the organs arising from the tract. From these three layers—**ectoderm mesoderm,** and **endoderm**—develop all the tissues of the body as well as the complex organs, which are composed of several types of tissue (Figure 1.11).

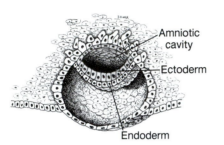

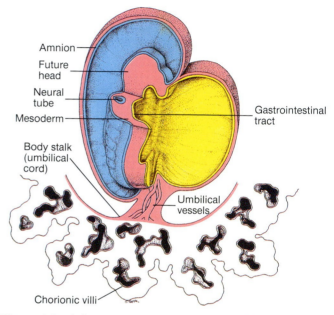

Figure 1.8 *A second small cavity lined with ectoderm develops (amniotic cavity). The other cavity (yolk sac) is lined with endoderm. The two cell layers contact in the center to form an area of ectoderm and endoderm (embryonic disc).*

Figure 1.9 *A three-week human embryo, viewed from the ventral aspect, illustrating an elongating gastrointestinal tube and dorsally located neural tube.*

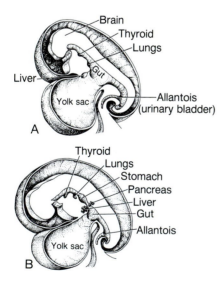

Figure 1.10 *Further development of the gastrointestinal tract at A, four and one-half weeks and B, five weeks. Note the appearance of the outpouchings of tube that will form the organs associated with gastrointestinal tract.*

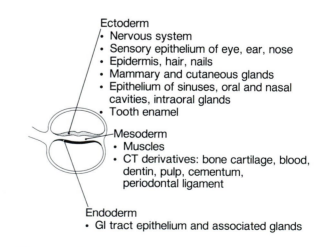

Ectoderm
- Nervous system
- Sensory epithelium of eye, ear, nose
- Epidermis, hair, nails
- Mammary and cutaneous glands
- Epithelium of sinuses, oral and nasal cavities, intraoral glands
- Tooth enamel

Mesoderm
- Muscles
- CT derivatives: bone cartilage, blood, dentin, pulp, cementum, periodontal ligament

Endoderm
- GI tract epithelium and associated glands

Figure 1.11 *Derivatives of ectoderm, mesoderm, and endoderm germ layers.*

■ Development of Human Tissues

Epithelial Structures and Derivatives

The skin is of dual origin, having an **epidermis,** a surface cell layer that develops from the surface ectodermal cells, and a **dermis,** which arises from the underlying mesoderm. The dermis originally comes from the **somites,** the masses of mesoderm that lie on either side of the neural tube (Figure 1.12). This mesoderm gives rise to both the dermis of the epithelium and the visceral mesoderm that covers the yolk sac and later becomes the gastrointestinal tract (Figure 1.12). Therefore, all the muscles functioning in peristalsis of the intestines arise from this mesoderm.

Initially, the embryo is covered with a single layer of ectodermal cells (Figure 1.13*A*.). By 11 to 12 weeks, this ectodermal layer or epithelium thickens into four layers. The basal layer of cells gives rise to the more superficial cells of the epithelium (Figure 1.13*B*). Later, **melanocytes** invade and pigment the skin (Figure 1.13*B*). At birth, the skin may show varying degrees of keratinization. Hair;

mammary, sebaceous, and salivary glands; teeth, and nails all develop from a combination of epidermal and dermal cells. This occurs when epithelial cells proliferate, invade the underlying dermis, and finally differentiate into glands or teeth, with both the epidermis and dermis contributing to each of these structures.

■ Clinical Comment

Environmental teratogens may affect the development of normal cells, tissues, organs, or organ systems. However, it is considerably less damaging to life and body function when a defect occurs in the normal development of a group of cells rather than in an organ or organ system. With a smaller and less complex maldevelopment, a less extensive problem is created. This developmental process is also related to timing, and when tissues begin to differentiate in the embryonic period (four to eight) weeks, they are the most susceptible to defective development.

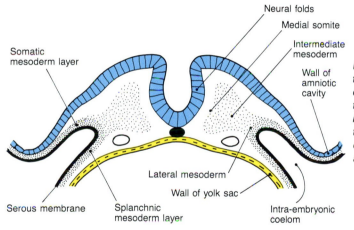

Somatic mesoderm layer

Neural folds

Medial somite

Intermediate mesoderm

Wall of amniotic cavity

Lateral mesoderm

Wall of yolk sac

Serous membrane

Splanchnic mesoderm layer

Intra-embryonic coelom

Figure 1.12 *The neural folds and somites in transverse section at approximately 20 days after conception. The medial somite, or mesoderm, forms the axial skeletal surrounding the neural tube. The intermediate mesoderm forms the striated muscle of the body, and the lateral mesoderm forms the dermis of the epithelium of the body wall (somatic) and of the gastrointestinal tract (splanchnic).*

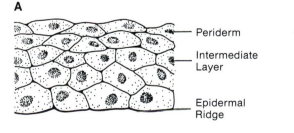

A

Periderm

Intermediate Layer

Epidermal Ridge

B

Stratum Corneum

Stratum Lucidum

Stratum Granulosum

Stratum Spinosum

Stratum Germinatum

Melanocyte

Dermis

Figure 1.13 *Development of skin **A,** at four weeks and **B,** 36 weeks. Initial layer of epithelial cells thickens into multiple layers, and the underlying connective tissue becomes the dermis. Dermis and epithelium combine to become skin.*

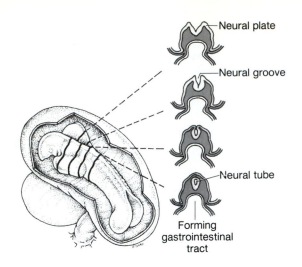

Figure 1.14   Left, *Dorsal view of the closing neural tube of a three-week human embryo. Note closure occurs initially in dorsal central area and then anteriorly and posteriorly.* Right, *Transverse sections of neural folds appear anteriorly, and those of the closed neural tube are in the midregion.*

Figure 1.15   *Development of the cranial nerves at* **A,** *three weeks,* **B,** *four weeks,* **C,** *five weeks, and* **D,** *six weeks. At three weeks, the forebrain has enlarged and the sensory vesicles are laterally located. At four and five weeks, the forebrain has bent forward, and cranial nerves have grown into tissues they innervate. At six weeks, anterior brain has enlarged and bent back on the posteriorly located cerebellum.*

Nervous System

The neural folds appear during the third prenatal week. The lateral edges of the neural plate then begin to elevate as folds that arise dorsally (Figure 1.9). These folds represent the first change in shape of the embryo's body from the flat sheet of cells described earlier (Figure 1.8). These folds contact in the midline, first in the cervical region, and then the neural tube closes both anteriorly and posteriorly (Figure 1.14). When the anterior tube closes, it shows three dilations that form the primary brain vesicles—the **forebrain, midbrain,** and **hindbrain** (Figure 1.15*A*). The neural tube then bends forward just behind the midbrain and backward behind the hindbrain (Figure 1.15*C* and *D*). The **cerebral hemispheres** develop from the forebrain. The midbrain is a pathway from the cerebral cortex to centers in the **pons** and **cerebellum** in the hindbrain. The fifth cranial nerve develops in the midbrain (Figure 1.15*B* to *D*). The cerebral hemispheres of the forebrain develop into the **frontal, temporal,** and **occipital lobes.**

The ventricles of the brain are continuous and connect posteriorly with the spinal cord. The walls of the neural tube are lined with neuroepithelium. As these cells proliferate, they differentiate into **neuroblasts,** which become the white and gray matter of the spinal cord. Neuroblasts are primitive nerve cells that develop into adult nerve cells, the **neurons.** These cells do not divide further. Along the surface of the developing brain and spinal cord, neural crest cells form the sensory system of the dorsal root ganglia of the cranial and spinal nerves (Figure 1.16). The neural crest cells also contribute to tissues of the face, such as cartilages, bones, muscles, teeth, and ligaments.

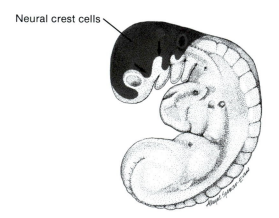

Figure 1.16   *Neural crest cells migrating from surface of neural tube ventrally to contribute to the developing face.*

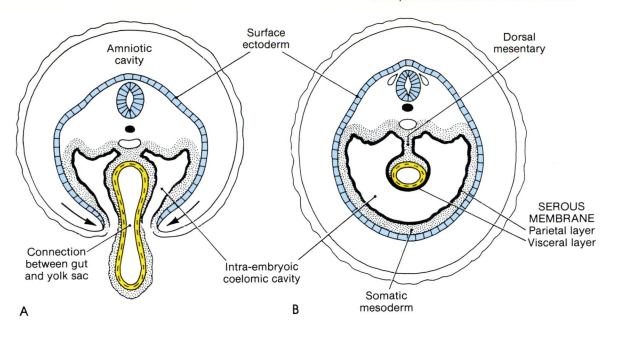

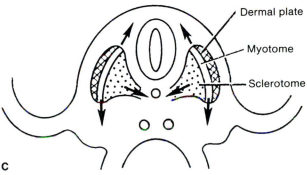

Figure 1.17 **A** and **B,** *Cross-sections of an embryo illustrating how yolk sac is incorporated into the elongating body as a gastrointestinal tube, and the elongating neural tube and enlarging brain at four weeks.* **C,** *The contribution of the somite to cartilage support of spinal column (the sclerotome). The muscles also arise from myotome (intermediate mesoderm) and dermal contribution (lateral mesoderm) to dermis of the body wall and gastrointestinal tube.*

Connective Tissue

Connective Tissue Proper

Connective tissue develops from the somites as fibroblasts, migrating from either side of the neural tube (Figure 1.12). Early in formation, the ventromedial part of the somite differentiates into the **sclerotome;** the dorsolateral part becomes the **dermatome,** and a third division is the intermediate mesoderm or **myotome.** The medial sclerotome portion differentiates into **mesenchymal cells,** which become **osteoblasts, chondroblasts,** and **fibroblasts.** From these cells, a large part of the embryonic

skeleton develops. Cells of the dermatome part of the somite form the dermis, the subcutaneous tissue, and **visceral mesoderm,** which supports the endoderm of the gastrointestinal tract (Figure 1.17A to C). From the third part, the myotome develops muscle, such as striated muscles of the body and limbs and the smooth muscle of the gastrointestinal tract, as well as a system of mesenteries that stabilize and support this tube (Figure 1.17). Also, connective tissue arises from the somites, providing supporting connective tissues, bones, cartilage, tendons, and ligaments. The tendons connect the muscles to the skeleton as they develop. Connective tissue also functions as capsules of glands and the supporting tissues within them.

Cartilage and Bone

The initial skeletal component in the embryo is **cartilage.** Cartilage cells arise from the sclerotome of the somites and migrate to surround the notochord and spinal cord forming the spinal column (Figure 1.17C). The skeleton develops in the same segmental pattern as do the muscles (Figures 1.18 and 1.21). Chondroblasts also form cartilage in the appendages, the cranium, and the face, first appearing in the fifth prenatal week. Cartilage cells undergo both **appositional** (exogenous) and **interstitial** (endogenous) growth (Figure 1.18B). Apposition of new layers of cartilage occurs on the surface of cartilage, and interstitial growth

involves the proliferation and expansion of the cells within the matrix (Figure 1.18B). Very rapidly, a supportive cartilage skeleton is produced to support the soft tissues of the growing embryo. Later, most of this same cartilage skeleton is replaced by bone, which offers more rigidity and strength as the muscles then attach to this skeleton, making movement possible (Figure 1.18C). Most cartilage appears clear and glasslike and is called **hyaline cartilage.** Cartilage may also contain elastic or fibrous tissue and is termed **elastic** or **fibrous cartilage.** The intervertebral discs, for example, are elastic cartilage, and the external ear contains fibrous cartilage. Cartilage combines the properties of elasticity and strength in these tissues.

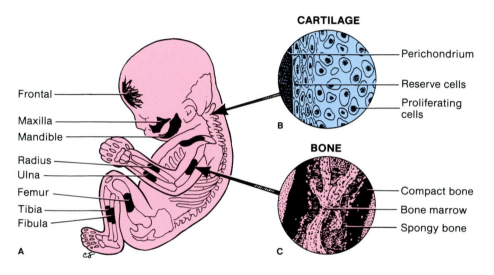

Figure 1.18   **A,** *Embryo's skeleton illustrating development of cartilage and bones.* **B,** *Cartilage development by both surface apposition and internal interstitial growth.* **C,** *Endochondral bone development in shaft of long bone.*

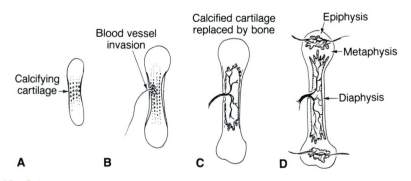

Figure 1.19   *Schematic diagram of endochondral ossification as seen in long bones of the body.* **A,** *Original hyaline cartilage is calcified in center.* **B,** *A blood vessel invades center of shaft.* **C,** *Marrow space appears in center of shaft as bone forms around it.* **D,** *Bone formation continues in shaft, and secondary ossification sites occur in the heads (epiphysis) of long bones. Disc of cartilage remains between bone forming in the head and shaft of (epiphyseal) bone.*

Bone replaces cartilage by a process termed **endochondral** bone development (Figure 1.19). In this case, a small blood vessel enters the cartilage shaft, the cartilage disintegrates in the center, and a marrow space is formed (Figure 1.19*B*). New bone develops on the surface of cartilage spicules that border the marrow space (Figure 1.19*C*.). During the growth period, a developing cartilage disc remains in the neck of each long bone and bone forms on either side. This disc is known as the **epiphyseal line** (Figure 1.19). The line allows for continued development of new cartilage and bone at this disc and thus provides for an increase in length of the long bone. Development occurs as new cartilage forms within the epiphyseal line by interstitial growth. New bone forms along the margins of the cartilage of the epiphyseal line. Later cartilage is limited to the covering of the heads of long bones, the nasal septum, the ears, and a few other sites.

Direct transformation of connective tissue into bone may also take place. In this case, collagen fibers in the connective tissue organize into a closely knit meshwork, and this matrix gradually calcifies into bone by a process called **intramembranous bone formation** (membranous bone formation) (Figure 1.20). The bones of the face and cranium are developed in this manner.

Muscle

By the tenth prenatal week, muscle cells (myoblasts) have begun migrating from the myotome portion of the somites, following a segmental pattern, similar to that of the bony skeleton (Figures 1.18 and 1.21). They gradually differentiate into elongated, multinucleated muscle fibers, which are specialized cells with the property of contractility. In this manner, muscle is able to provide motion on the basis of structural and functional characteristics.

Muscle is divided into three types: skeletal, smooth, and cardiac. Later, these skeletal muscles lose their segmental pattern of development as they acquire insertion on skeletal elements. These muscle fibers become the **striated voluntary muscles,** which divide into groups that supply the dorsal and ventral parts of the limbs and provide both the deep and the superficial muscle fibers (Figure 1.22). These muscles are called striated because they have lines, which are the contraction sites, across them. This causes the muscles to function.

Muscle cells also migrate to the gastrointestinal tract, support the trachea, bronchi, urogenital tract, and larger blood vessels. These muscle cells develop and become oriented in the direction in which their contractility will be exerted. They are termed **smooth muscle cells.** These muscle cells are under the control of the autonomic nervous system and not under conscious control as are skeletal muscles. The blood vessels that develop in the head region, limbs, and body wall gain their muscular coat from local mysenchyme.

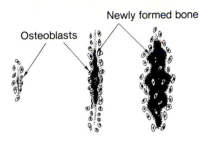

Figure 1.20 *Membranous bone formation that takes place in connective tissue. Initial membranous sites grow by apposition of new bone on their surfaces.*

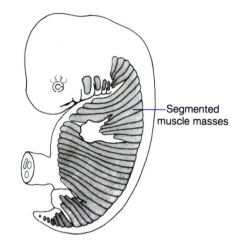

Figure 1.21 *Schematic diagram of primitive myotome in skeletal muscle formation in embryo.*

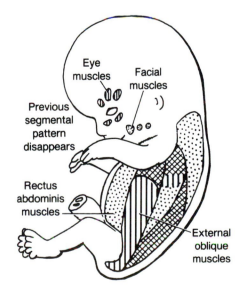

Figure 1.22 *Differentiation of skeletal muscle by enlargement of fibers and attachment to bony skeleton to become functional units.*

Cardiovascular System

The cardiovascular system originates from cells termed **angioblasts,** which arise from **angiogenic clusters** located in the walls of the yolk sac during the third week of prenatal life (Figure 1.23). As these cells separate into clusters, the outer cells organize into a series of elongating tubes, and the inner cells become blood cells (Figure 1.24). Nutrition moves from the yolk sac to the embryo through this developing **vitelline** vascular system for a short time (Figure 1.25). The yolk sac contains nutriment that briefly supplies the embryo. However, vitelline vessels conduct blood from the yolk sac to the embryo. The entire blood vascular system within the embryo is created in the same manner, with longitudinal growth of vessels and the appearance of blood cells within them. As vessels begin to develop in the embryo, they in turn form a vascular network connected to the placenta. Since it traverses the umbilical cord, this network is termed the **umbilical system** (Figure 1.25). Through this umbilical system, nutrition and oxygen are conducted to the embryo, and carbon dioxide and wastes to the placenta. By the fourth prenatal week, the heart begins to beat. This vascular system takes over the function as the vitelline system expires because the yolk sac lacks any further contribution (Figure 1.25).

Other mesenchymal cells migrate into the pericardial area to function in the development of the heart tubes, and these cells later differentiate into cardiac muscle. Two angiogenic cell clusters initially give rise to two straight bilat-eral endocardial heart tubes, which fuse during the third week. They then enlarge and bend back upon themselves (Figure 1.26). As the great vessels that bring blood to the heart enlarge and become more extensive, the heart enlarges and internal partitioning of the heart begins. An opening remains between the atria (foramen ovale) until birth, however. As the heart tube enlarges and twists in development, the strands of muscle take on the arrangement of parallel fibers. Like striated muscle, these fibers develop transverse markings termed **intercalated discs.** The myofibrils on either side of these discs exert contraction through the interaction of these many cells. Cardiac muscle thus is not under conscious control and begins to beat in the fourth prenatal week. The umbilical circulation then becomes active in transport of oxygen and nutrition from the placenta.

■ Clinical Comment

Aging is the process in which the capacity for replacement of worn-out cells is diminished. A possible result can be seen in the loss or graying of the hair. Also, aging is seen as a diminution of bone, muscle, and other supportive tissue, resulting in decreased function. Disease is usually another factor contributing to this process of tissue modification or destruction. For example, disease may modify the shape of bones, and then in aging of their structure and function is further diminished.

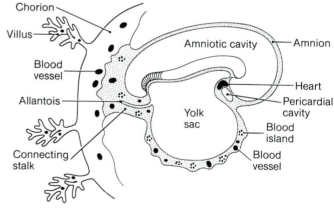

Figure 1.23 *Origin of blood cells and blood vessels in walls of yolk sac, placenta, and body stalk in two and one-half-week-old embryo.*

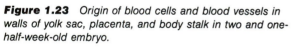

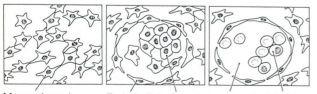

Mesenchymal cells   Endothelial cells   Blood island   Lumen of primitive blood vessel   Primitive blood cell

Figure 1.24 *Appearance of blood islands from mesenchymal cells in location noted in Figure 1.23. The more peripheral cells form capillaries, and the inner cells form red blood cells. The tubes (capillaries) then lengthen.*

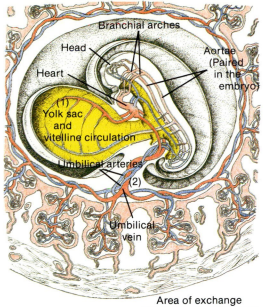

Figure 1.25 *Development of blood vascular system in embryo. (1) In the yolk sac, the vitelline circulation develops, persisting for only a few weeks until this nutritional source is exhausted. (2) Umbilical system develops in umbilical cord and supplies embryo and fetus with oxygen and nutrients until birth.*

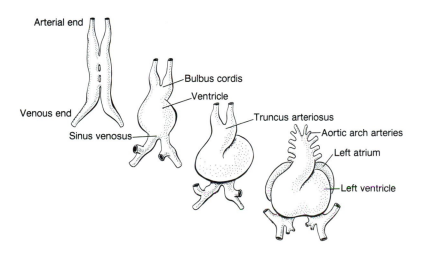

Figure 1.26 *Development of the four-chamber heart from the fusion of two lateral endocardiac heart tubes. There is lateral folding of the tubes into a single tube, which is next divided by internal septa into a four-chamber heart.*

■ Self-Evaluation Questions

1. What is the smallest unit of structure and its eight functions in the body?
2. Name and give the functions of the structures found in the cell cytoplasm.
3. Name and discuss cells that do not undergo cell division.
4. Define the cell cycle, mitosis, and meiosis. What activities occur in the G1 and G2 phases?
5. Describe the embryonic disc's appearance in the third and fourth prenatal weeks.
6. Define the three periods of prenatal development.
7. What is the significance of angiogenic cluster and the vitelline and umbilical vascular systems?
8. What develops from the foregut, midgut, and hindgut (gastrointestinal tract)?
9. Name the structure and function of the different types of muscles.
10. Name and describe the three types of cartilage and two types of bone.

■ Acknowledgments

Dr. N.M. Elnesr contributed to Chapter 1, General Human Development, in Avery, J.K., ed., *Oral Development and Histology,* Toronto: B.C. Decker, 1988. With appreciation, some of the comments and figures have been used in this text.

■ Suggested Reading

Avery, J.K., ed. Oral development and histology. Toronto: B.C. Decker, 1988.

Moore, K.L. The developing human, 2nd ed. Philadelphia: W.B. Saunders, 1977.

Sadler, T., ed. Langman's medical embryology, 5th ed. Baltimore: Williams & Wilkins, 1985.

Sperber, G.H. Craniofacial embryology, 4th ed. London: Butterworth, 1989.

Tortora, G.J. Principles of human anatomy, 5th ed. New York: Harper & Row, 1989.

2 Structure and Function of Cells, Tissues, and Organs

■ Overview

This chapter describes the structure and function of the body's primary tissues: epithelial, neural, connective, and muscle. In Chapter 1, the development of these tissues was presented.

This chapter first describes the epithelial tissues as to cell type, cell structure, and location and function in the body. Simple squamous epithelium lines the blood vascular and respiratory systems, the kidney, most glands, and the intestine. Stratified squamous epithelium, on the other hand, is limited to the lining of the mouth, pharynx, larynx and part of the urinary bladder.

Neural tissue is the next type considered; both the central nervous system, composed of the brain and spinal cord, and the nerves and ganglia of the peripheral nervous system are discussed. The basic structural unit of the nervous system, the neuron, along with its supporting neuroglia cells forms a communication network. The two properties of a neuron are irritability and conductivity, which enable neurons to react and respond to stimuli.

The third type discussed is connective tissue, characterized by its abundant matrix, composed of fibers and amorphous ground substance. These tissues are classified according to associated cells, fibers, and location and function. Connective tissue proper consists of loose and dense connective tissue and loose tissue with special properties. Two other specialized types of connective tissue are cartilage and bone. Three types of cartilage are described—hyaline, elastic, and fibrous—followed by both cancellous (spongy) and compact (dense) bone. The fourth type of connective tissue is blood and lymph.

Finally the three types of muscle—striated voluntary, smooth involuntary, and cardiac—are described according to cell shape and matrix and their functions in the body.

Nine organ systems are then described to illustrate how tissues combine to carry out specialized functions in the human body. Correlative tables are provided to assist in the understanding of this information.

■ *Epithelial Tissue*

Epithelial tissue is composed of closely packed sheets of cells covering the external surface and internal cavities of the body and the tubes leading to glands or follicles that develop from the surface or internal epithelium. Epithelial cells form membranes that are composed of closely associated cells with little intercellular substance between them.

The **epidermis** and **dermis** constitute the skin. The epidermis, which is a form of epithelium, rests on a basement membrane that separates it from the connective tissue termed dermis.

Since epithelium does not contain blood vessels, it depends on vessels located in the connective tissue that are in close proximity. Most epithelium has the capability of cell renewal by mitosis, and the rate of renewal is dependent on the location of the epithelium in the body. For example, human buccal mucosa changes in 10 to 14 days, whereas the junctional epithelium of the gingiva renews in 4 to 6 days.

Epithelium is described by cell shape, and their arrangement is in one or more layers. Some cells form a single layer known as **simple epithelium.** Epithelium with all cells in contact with the basal lamina, but not with the surface, is known as pseudostratified. The type consisting of several layers of cells with only the basal cells in contact with the basal lamina is known as **stratified epithelium** (Figure 2.1). Further modifications are based on the cell shape. Epithelial membranes function in one or more of the processes of absorption, contractility, digestion, excretion, protection, secretion, and sensation. Table 2.1 shows the classification of epithelia by cell type, cell shape, cell modifications, and location and function.

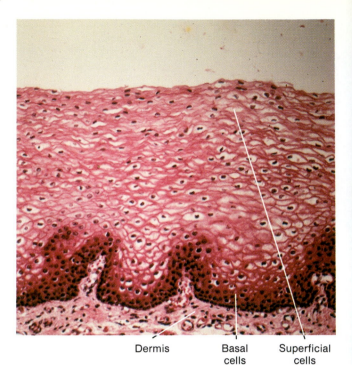

Dermis   Basal cells   Superficial cells

Figure 2.1 *Stratified squamous nonkeratinized epithelium from oral cavity. Observe multicellular layers. Darker-stained cells are basal cells, which are dividing to give rise to all of the more superficial cell layers. As they develop in basal layer, they migrate to surface. Dark cells lie adjacent to dermis, which contains the blood vessels that nourish the epithelium.*

■ *Neural Tissue*

A second tissue type is neural tissue, which constitutes the central and peripheral nervous systems. The **central nervous system** (CNS) is the control center of the nervous system and is composed of the brain and spinal cord. The brain is located in the cranium and continues into the spinal cord. It is formed of neuroepithelial cells, which are highly organized areas for reception and correlation. All sensation received anywhere in the body is relayed to the brain and spinal cord, where it is acted upon. Nerve processes that carry information and convey it from the peripheral nervous system in muscles and glands to the CNS are called the **afferent (sensory) system.** Other neurons that convey responses from the CNS to muscles and glands are located in the **efferent (motor) system.** These two systems are further divided into the **somatic** and **autonomic** nervous systems.

The somatic nervous system (soma) carries impulses to the voluntary muscles, such as the skeletal muscles, which are under conscious control. On the other hand, the efferent autonomic system carries impulses from the CNS to involuntary muscles such as the smooth and cardiac muscles and to all the glands. The viscera also receive most of their impulses from this system.

This system produces responses involuntarily and is further divided into the **sympathetic** and **parasympathetic** divisions. These two divisions modify each other: the sympathetic causes increased activity, and the autonomic modifies or decreases activity. Table 2.2 provides a summary of this system.

The nervous system carries out its numerous functions with only two principal types of cells: the **neuron** and **neuroglia** cells. Neurons are the nerve cells that carry out the function of the nervous system in reception of impulses and conduction and regulation of muscle and gland activity. Neuroglia cells are the supporting cells of the nervous system. Each neuron consists of three parts. The first is the **cell body** or **perikaryon,** which contains the nucleus, and the cytoplasm, which contains chromatophilic substance or **rough endoplasmic reticulum (RER).** The function of the

Table 2.1   Classification of Epithelia

Cell type	Cell shape	Cell modifications	Location and function
Simple			
1. Squamous			
a. Endothelial	Spindle-shaped		Lines heart, blood, and lymph vessels
b. Mesothelial	Oval to polygonal		Lines pleural, pericardial, and peritoneal cavities
2. Cuboidal	Cube-shaped	Cilia may appear.	Kidney, glands, respiratory passages
3. Columnar	Rodlike	Microvilli, cilia may appear.	Most glands, small intestines, respiratory passages
4. Pseudostratified	Rodlike with thin section	Cilia, stereocilia	Respiratory passages, male reproductive organs
Stratified			
1. Squamous	Polyhedral	Intercellular bridges	Covering of the body, mouth, pharynx, vagina
2. Columnar	Columnar cells on cuboidal or columnar on columnar		Oropharynx, larynx
3. Transitional	Cube- to pear-shaped	Distention causes cell flattening.	Urinary passages and bladder

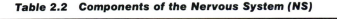

Table 2.2   Components of the Nervous System (NS)

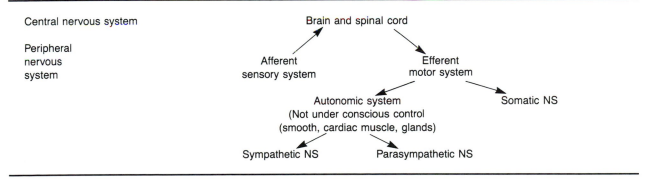

RER, as with other cells, is protein synthesis. Proteins travel from the perikaryon into the axon, which is the second part of the cell. The axon is a long, thin singular process, which varies in length from a few millimeters to several feet or more. It conducts nerve impulses away from the nerve cell body. The axon terminates by branching into axon terminals (synaptic end bulbs) (Figure 2.2). Axons outside the CNS are protected and insulated by a myelin sheath, which is a multilayer of phospholipid. This myelin is produced by the neurolemmocytes (Schwann's cells). The third component of the neuron is the **dendrite,** usually multiple, which functions to receive and conduct impulses to the cell body (Figure 2.2).

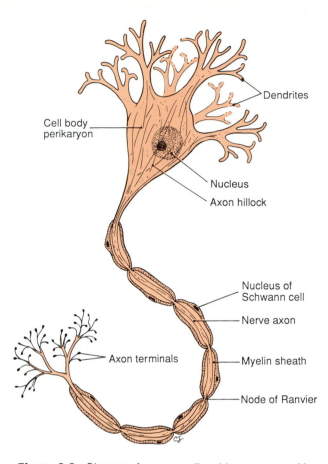

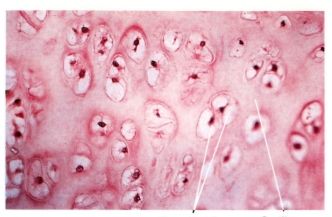

Chondrocytes   Cartilage
                      matrix

Figure 2.3 *Section of hyaline cartilage found in thyroid or tracheal cartilages. Large cells (chondrocytes) can be seen surrounded by a homogenous-appearing cartilage matrix. Only dark-stained nucleoli can be seen, since cytoplasm of the cells is faintly stained. Cells exist in lacunae, which are open spaces in the matrix. Some cells have divided, and two cells appear in the same or adjacent lacunae.*

Figure 2.2 *Diagram of a nerve cell and its processes. Myelin insulates nerve axon and is produced by Schwann cells. Impulses travel from cell body to axon terminals where they may contact dendrites of an adjacent nerve cell.*

In addition to the neuron, there are cells that carry out the functions of support, termed neuroepithelial cells. These are 5 to 10 times more numerous than neurons. Neuroepithelial cells protect and support nerve cells, and some of these cells are even phagocytic, ingesting bacteria.

The brain continues into the spinal cord, which is within the vertebral canal. This canal is a cylindrical space extending from the brain to the lumbar vertebrae. It is composed of 31 segments, each giving rise to spinal nerves. The spinal cord conveys impulses from the peripheral nervous system to the brain and from the brain to the periphery.

■ Connective Tissue

This tissue varies as to its proportion of cells, fibers, and intercellular substance and its location in the body. Connective tissue proper is classified in structure as **loose, dense,** or **loose connective tissue with special properties.** Two other types of connective tissue are the skeletal tissues—cartilage and bone. There are three types of cartilage—**hyaline** (Figure 2.3), **elastic,** and **fibrous** (Figure

2.4). Bone is classified according to its structure as **compact** (dense) or **cancellous** (spongy) (Figures 2.5 to 2.7). The fourth type of connective tissue is blood and lymph (Figure 2.8). Each type of connective tissue has specific associated cells and fibers, with special functions and locations in the body. This tissue is classified in Table 2.3 and seen in Figures 2.3 to 2.5.

■ Clinical Comment

Knowledge of bone formation and resorption is clinically important in the understanding of orthodontic tooth movement or in physiologic mesial drift. Bone removal in the direction of tooth movement is the initial step in the process. This is gained by pressure of the tooth on the alveolar bone. This bone is responsive and resorption occurs. Osteoclasts mobilize in a short time and bone removal begins. As the tooth begins to move, the periodontal fibers pull on the opposite surface of the root, stimulating bone formation in the space from where the tooth moved.

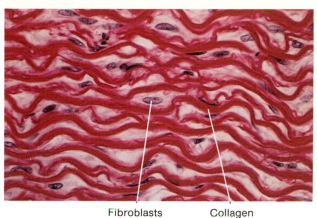

Fibroblasts   Collagen
fibers

Figure 2.4 *Appearance of dense, irregular connective tissue. Large bundles of collagen fibers appear in longitudinal section with a few pale-stained fibroblasts interspersed between them. Under the electron microscope the faint banding of these collagen fibers may be seen.*

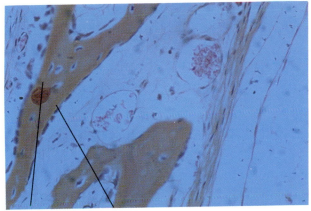

Bone   Osteoblasts
matrix

Figure 2.6 *Appearance of cancellous bone. If this were newly forming intramembranous bone, there would be numerous osteoblasts on the surface of the trabeculae. A few elongated and flattened osteoblasts can be seen on the surface of bone trabeculae. Several thin-walled veins can be seen in the field as well as scattered connective tissue cells.*

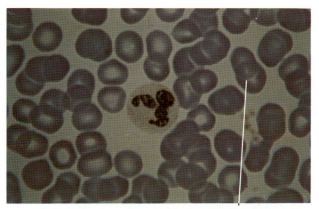

Erythrocytes

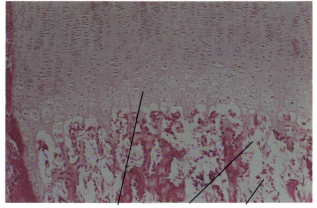

Cartilage   Bone   Bone
marrow

Figure 2.5 *Developing endochondral bone matrix. Where bone spicules can be seen below and cartilage above, is area of transition of cartilage into bone. The hyaline cartilage above becomes calcified and undergoes a breakdown. Across the field, spicules of bone are formed in the center of a long bone, called the bone marrow. New cartilage also forms in the area shown at top of photo, which maintains the cartilage, until growth is complete.*

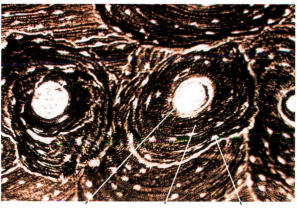

Haversian   Concentric   Lacunae
canals   lamellae

Figure 2.7 *Compact bone in transverse section illustrating haversian systems. Haversian canals are surrounded by concentric lamellae with (white) lacunae between the lamellae. If this were living bone, the lacunae would contain osteocytes. Between haversian systems are other lamellae, called interstitial lamellae, which are remains of earlier remodeling of a haversian system.*

Figure 2.8 *This blood smear simulates the appearance of circulating blood by showing the numerous red blood cells (erythrocytes) and occasional white blood cells (neutrophils). Observe comparative size of the cells. Red (pink) blood cells are white in the center since they are biconcave discs. They are thin and transparent when dried, as in this preparation.*

Table 2.3   Classification of Connective Tissue

Tissue type	Associated cells	Fibers		Location and function
1. Connective tissue proper				
A. Loose connective tissue	Fibroblasts, macrophages, mast cells	Yellow elastic White collagen		Fascia, superficial and deep; organ framework support
B. Dense connective tissue				
1. Dense regular	Fibroblasts, macrophages	White fibrous		Tendons, ligaments; muscle to bone attachment
2. Dense irregular	Fibroblasts, macrophages	Mostly white fibrous, elastic and reticular fibers		Sheets, dermis, some sternum, capsules; support of organs
C. Loose connective tissue with special properties				
1. Mucous connective tissue	Stellate fibroblasts	Collagenous		Umbilical and vocal cords; support
2. Elastic tissue	Fibroblasts	Yellow elastic		Ligamenta nuchae, vocal cords; support
3. Reticular tissue	Reticular cells	Fine reticular		Framework of lymph node and spleen
4. Adipose tissue	Fat cells	None		Scattered in all loose connective tissue and in deposits
5. Pigment tissue	Melanoblasts	None		Corium of dark skin Choroid and iris of eye
2. Cartilage				
A. Hyaline cartilage	Chondrocytes	Fine collagenous fibers		Articular and nasal cartilages, trachea, bronchi; support
B. Elastic cartilage	Chondrocytes	Elastic, collagenous		External ear, eustachian tube, epiglottis; support
C. Fibrous cartilage	Chondrocytes	Collagenous (dense)		Intervertebral discs; support
3. Bone				
A. Spongy or cancellous	Osteocytes, osteoblasts osteoclasts	Collagenous		Center of long bones
B. Compact or dense	Osteocytes, osteoclasts, osteoblasts	Collagenous		Outer shaft of bones
4. Blood and lymph	Erythrocytes, leukocytes			Blood vascular and lymphatic systems

■ Clinical Comment

One clinically relevant example of the interaction of epithelium, connective tissue, blood vascular tissue, and bone occurs in the healing of an oral wound such as a tooth socket. Initially, a blood clot fills the socket; after a few days, fibroblasts appear in the clot, and surface epithelial cells proliferate to close the wound. During the second week, a vascular network and collagen fibers organize in the socket. This is called granulation tissue. In the third week, organization of fibers and vessels continues, the clot is forced to the surface, and epithelial cells close the wound under the clot. Fine trabeculae of bone then begin organizing in the socket, and the process continues until healing is complete.

■ Muscle Tissue

There are three different types of muscle: **skeletal** (Figure 2.9), **smooth** (Figure 2.10), and **cardiac** (Figure 2.11). Each muscle type has its own characteristic. Involuntary movement, for example, is representative of cardiac and smooth muscle. This means that the muscle is under the control of the body and not under the individual's voluntary control. Skeletal, or striated, muscle movement, however, is under voluntary control, and this movement represents all the muscles of the body appendages and trunk.

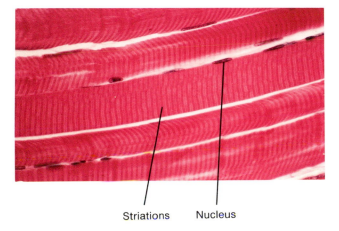

Striations   Nucleus

Figure 2.9 *Skeletal muscle fibers in longitudinal section. Cross-striations are seen as alternating light and dark bands, indicating sites of contraction of fibers. Each large fiber contains a number of nuclei located on periphery. These are muscle fibers of arms, legs, and body wall and are controlled voluntarily by humans.*

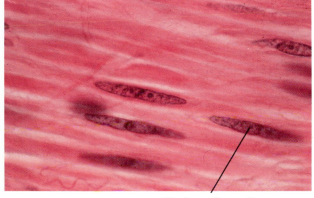

Nucleus of smooth muscle cell

Figure 2.10 *Smooth muscle fibers in longitudinal section; can be compared to skeletal muscle. Fibers are spindle-shaped, and the large, elongated nucleus is in center of the fiber. Small amounts of connective tissue surround the fibers. This muscle surrounds the gastrointestinal tract and blood vessels. It is controlled involuntarily.*

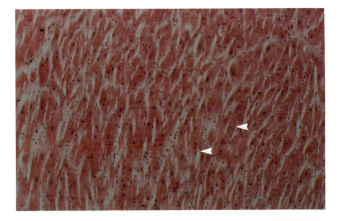

Figure 2.11 *Section of cardiac muscle found in the heart wall. Muscle fibers appear striated and are similar to skeletal muscle fibers except some fibers branch (arrows). The nuclei of these fibers are located centrally, as seen in smooth muscle, and the area at the ends of the nuclei are pale staining.*

Table 2.4   Classification of Muscle

Type	Cell shape	Diagrams	Location
A. Skeletal (Skeletal wall, voluntary)	Very long multinucleated fiber with cross-striations composed of actin (thin) anbd myosin (thick) components.		To the bony skeleton or fascia, limbs and body, pharynx, upper esophagus
B. Smooth Visceral, involuntary	Spindle-shaped fibers with a single elongated nucleus and myofilaments. Nuclei located in center of fiber.		In hollow organs, wall of intestines, ducts of glands, and blood vessels
C. Cardiac muscle Striated, involuntary	Long cross-striated fibers that branch and contain intercalated discs (junctional complexes). Some muscle fibers are specialized to conduct impulses: Purkinje's fibers. Nuclei in center of fiber.		Wall of heart and major veins opening into the heart

Some features of muscle are common to all types. For example, each muscle fiber is covered with **perimysium,** and the entire muscle is covered with **epimysium.** The contractile elements of muscle are actin and myosin, which are arranged differently in each type of muscle. The property common to all muscle types is the ability to contract. A description of the muscle types, their location, and the cells that function within each is presented in Table 2.4.

■ Organ Systems

Organ systems comprise those tissues in the body that are functionally integrated and designed to carry out specific functions. They are first composed of cells and their products, which may be diverse in nature but function as a unit. Figure 2.12 is a diagram of the organ systems. There are nine organ systems, which are described as follows.

Integumentary or Skin System.   This is the largest organ composed of epidermis, dermis, connective tissue, and muscle. This system has the following functions: protection to keep out foreign materials, sensation by neural receptors in the dermis, temperature control, and excretion of waste by sweat glands.

Digestive System.   The digestive system is composed of four layers, including loose connective tissue, muscle, connective tissue, and epithelium. It also consists of glands such as the salivary glands, liver, and pancreas, which empty their secretions into this tube. The function of the digestive system is to transform, adsorb, and excrete food (Figures 2.13 and 2.14).

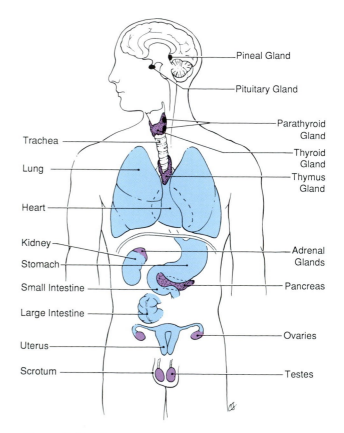

Figure 2.12   *Diagram of human body showing location of glands on right side of the body and the organs on the left side.*

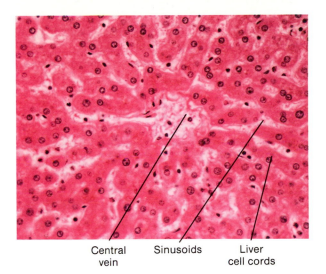

Central vein   Sinusoids   Liver cell cords

Figure 2.13 *Section of liver tissue illustrating liver cell cords radiating from central vein. Blood filters from periphery of each liver (hepatic) lobule. This organ filters the blood and provides a storage area. Spaces between the cell cords are termed sinusoids. Note the large oval nuclei of liver cells.*

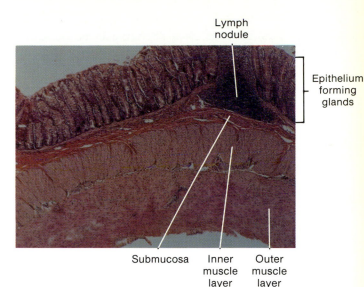

Lymph nodule

Epithelium forming glands

Submucosa   Inner muscle layer   Outer muscle layer

Figure 2.14 *Section of a colon illustrating epithelium forming deep glands in the mucosa. Supported by connective tissue, lymph nodules are seen as dense aggregations of lymphocytes in this layer of glands. Beneath this is the submucosa made up of connective tissue containing arteries, veins, capillaries, and nerves. Below this zone are the muscular layers; the inner layer is longitudinal and the outer circular. On the surface of the intestine is thin connective tissue, the serosal layer.*

Respiratory System. This system includes the nasal passages, trachea, bronchi, and lungs proper, all of which function in respiration. The respiratory tract is lined with epithelia that are taller near the bronchi and trachea and shorter near the terminal air sacs, which are effective in the exchange of oxygen and carbon dioxide.

Lymphatic System. This system includes the thymus, spleen, tonsils, lymph nodes, and lymphatic nodules located in various parts of the digestive system. The system produces antibodies against foreign substances, especially proteins and bacteria.

Vascular System. This system includes the heart and all arteries, veins, and capillaries. They function to produce and circulate blood, to carry various gases to all areas of the body, and to eliminate foreign substances by phagocytosis. Arteries have a layer of elastic connective tissue known as internal elastic lamina and a thick muscular layer that makes the arteries appear round in a histologic section. Veins are thin-walled, have little muscle, and may appear flattened.

Endocrine Systems. This system includes the thyroid and parathyroid glands, pituitary gland, ovaries, testes, pancreas, and adrenal medulla. A basic function of these glands is to secrete hormones into the vascular circulation, which in turn acts on target cells through the second-messenger cyclic adenosine monophosphate (cAMP).

Urinary System. The urinary system is composed of the kidneys, ureters, bladder, and an external urinary meatus. This system filters toxic and unneeded substances from the blood stream, concentrating and excreting them.

Reproductive System. The reproductive system includes the testes, ovaries, uterus, vagina, prostate, and seminal vesicles. The system produces eggs and sperm with half the chromosome complement by reduction division and meiosis. This allows fertilization of the egg by the sperm and provides a place for the egg to attach and develop.

Special Senses.   The sensory system includes the eyes, ears, and nose, all of which contain the four tissue types.

■ Clinical Comment

Oral infections may cause pain, tenderness, swelling, and enlarged local lymph nodes. Pain is due to the response of a nerve receptor to damage and then transmission to the brain, with corresponding efferent response to both autonomic and somatic systems. This results in a change in vascular tone, causing swelling. Lymph nodes enlarge as defense cells proliferate and become active, filtering and destroying the bacteria and their products in the local lymph nodes.

■ Self-Evaluation Questions

1. Describe the four types of loose connective tissue that have special properties.
2. Describe the two types of connective tissue proper.
3. Describe the three types of cartilage and their location in the body.
4. Describe cancellous and compact bone and the location of both types.
5. Describe the two types of muscle that have involuntary movement and their function.
6. What are the nonstratified epithelial cell types, and where are they located in the body?
7. Describe the location of stratified squamous and columnar epithelium.
8. Discuss the function of the autonomic nervous system.
9. Describe how the sympathetic and parasympathetic nervous systems work together.
10. Name and briefly describe each of the nine organ systems.

■ Suggested Reading

Fawcett, D.W. The cell, 2nd ed. Philadelphia: W.B. Saunders, 1981.

Kelly, D.E., Wood, R.L., and Enders, A.C. Bailey's textbook of microscopic anatomy, 18th ed. Baltimore: Williams & Wilkins, 1984.

Leeson, C.R., and Leeson, TS.: Textbook of histology, 5th ed. Philadelphia: W.B. Saunders, 1985.

Leeson, T.S., Leeson, C.R., and Paparo, A.A. Textbook/atlas of histology. Philadelphia: W.B. Saunders, 1988.

Tortora, G.J. Principles of human anatomy, 5th ed. New York: Harper & Row, 1989.

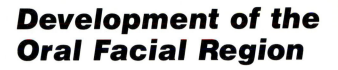

Development of the Oral Facial Region

■ Overview

This chapter concerns development and orientation of the tissues that form the human face and neck. During the fourth week of development, the human embryo consists of a flat disc that bends down at its extremity as the overlying brain expands and enlarges. This action pushes the heart beneath the brain. A pit develops in the midline between the brain above and the heart below, which becomes the oral cavity, or stomodeum (Figure 3.1). Beneath this cavity, the first **branchial arch,** termed the **mandibular arch,** forms, and the maxillary tissues that form the cheeks grow out of this first arch. Below the mandibular arch, four other branchial arches, or bars, appear during the fourth to seventh prenatal weeks. The second arch is called the **hyoid** (Figure 3.2). These parallel arches are important in the development of the face and neck, and each contains blood vessels, muscles, nerves, and skeletal elements. Aortic arch blood vessels, which course through each branchial arch from the heart below to the brain above, are important to craniofacial development. The first, second, and fifth of these vessels are transient. The third arch vessel quickly assumes the role of supplying the first and second arches. This vessel also transforms the vascular supply of the face from the **internal carotid** to the **external carotid.** Muscles arise in each of the branchial arches; the mandibular arch muscles become the muscles of mastication, and the second arch muscles become those of facial expression. The muscles of the third and fourth arches serve the throat. Nerves follow these muscles: the fifth nerve is in the first arch, the seventh in the second, the ninth in the third, the tenth in the fourth, and the eleventh in the fifth. Cartilages also appear in each arch: **Meckel's cartilage bar** is in the first, the **superior hyoid** in the second, the **inferior hyoid** in the third, and the **laryngeal cartilages** in the fourth. In addition, cartilages arise from the first arch and appear in the upper face. The **sense capsules** support the olfactory and auditory nerves and the upper face. The **cranial base** underlies and supports the brain.

All the creative events described in this chapter span just the short period of facial organization, which takes place from the fourth to the seventh weeks of gestation.

■ *Development of the Oropharynx*

The oropharynx is encompassed by the primitive oral cavity and the area of the foregut called the pharynx. The oral pit first appears in the fourth week of human development when the neural plate bends ventrally as the neural folds develop to form the forebrain (see Figure 3.1). This cephalocaudal bend pushes the heart ventrally, and the yolk sac then becomes enclosed as an elongating tube known as the foregut (Figure 3.1).

The deepening oral pocket then appears between the forebrain and heart. This pocket eventually becomes the oral cavity (Figure 3.2). At its deepest extent is the **oropharyngeal** membrane lining, which upon rupturing in the fifth week will open the oral cavity into the tubular foregut, soon to be the pharynx (Figures 3.3 and 3.4). Below this oral pit is a horizontal bar of tissue, the first branchial arch, which will form the mandible. The mandibular arch will grow lateral to the oral pit, developing the maxillary processes that form the cheeks.

The enlarging heart now becomes positioned below the mandibular arch in the thorax and begins beating at the end of this fourth week (Figure 3.3). Blood is then forced through these vessels in the branchial arches, which supply the face, neck, and brain. The forming face then grows away from the forebrain and presses against the chest and heart.

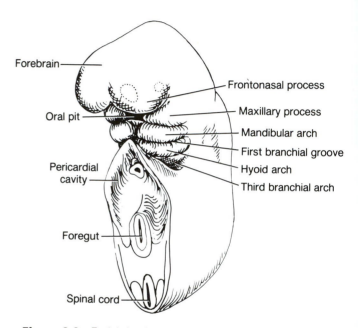

Figure 3.2 *Facial development in fourth prenatal week. Observe oral pit with facial primordia surrounding it. Note branchial arches and grooves. The heart develops in thorax.*

Figure 3.1 *Anterior embryonic disc bends inferiorly with growth and expansion of developing brain. This pushes the heart ventrally, and the oral pit (stomodeum) develops between the brain and heart.*

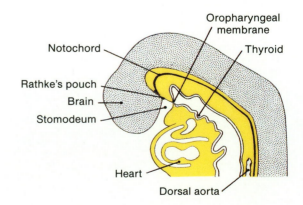

Figure 3.3 *Internal view of oral pit at three and one-half weeks. Observe oropharyngeal membrane separating oral and pharyngeal tubes. This membrane will soon rupture.*

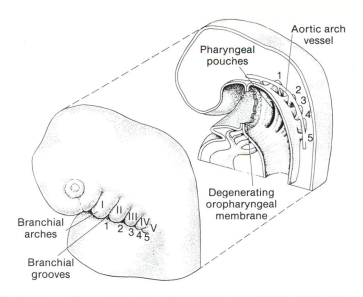

Figure 3.4 *Sagittal view of branchial arches with corresponding grooves behind each arch. The pharyngeal pouches are seen in pharynx. Vasculature of aortic arch leads from heart below dorsally to face.*

■ Development of the Branchial Arches

The branchial arches are so termed because they bend around the sides of the pharynx as bars of tissue. Each is separated by vertical grooves on the lateral sides of the neck, at the fifth week of human life. Within the pharynx, grooves called **pharyngeal pouches** separate each arch. These pouches match the branchial clefts on the external aspects of the neck (see Figure 3.4).

The five arches with their clefts resemble the embryonic gill slits of fish and amphibians. It is one of the many similarities between human embryos and other embryos during early development. The first arch is termed the mandibular arch, since it will later form the bony mandible, the associated muscles of mastication, nerves, and blood supply. The second, or hyoid, arch forms the facial muscles, vessels, and hyoid bone. The third, fourth, and fifth arches consist of paired right and left bars that are divided before they reach the midline by the presence of the bulging heart (see Figure 3.2). The arches get progressively smaller, anterior to posterior. The outer surface of each arch is covered with ectoderm, as is the inner surface of the first and the anterior part of the second, which is the epithelial lining of the oral cavity. The pharyngeal surface of the remaining four arches, however, is lined by endoderm, the same as the remainder of the gastrointestinal tract (Figure 3.4). In the core of each arch, the blood vessels, muscles, nerves, cartilages, and bones will differentiate; these are important in the development of the adult human face.

■ Clinical Comment

During the short span from the fourth to the seventh prenatal weeks, the face develops an environmental factor that could cause a branchial arch or facial defect likely to affect these tissues before the fourth week after conception. This is a time to be especially careful of irradiation and dietary, chemical, and stress-related factors.

Branchial Grooves and Pharyngeal Pouches

The first branchial groove deepens to become the **external auditory canal** leading to the middle ear. The membrane at the depth of this tube becomes the **tympanic membrane.** From the corresponding first pouch, the middle ear and eustachian tube develop. After the fifth week, no other branchial grooves are seen externally, as the second arch then grows caudally over the surface of the others to contact the fifth arch (Figure 3.5). This overgrowth obscures the other arches and grooves externally, though their internal structures play an important role in facial development.

The endodermal lining of the pharyngeal pouches differentiates into several important organs. The second pharyngeal pouch gives rise to the **palatine tonsils;** the third gives rise to the **inferior parathyroid** and **thymus;** the fourth gives rise to the **superior parathyroid;** and from the fifth develops the **ultimobranchial body** (Figure 3.5).

The palatine tonsils function in the development of lymphocytes, which are important in immunology of the body. The parathyroid glands regulate calcium balance throughout life. The thymus, located behind the sternum and between the lungs, is large at birth and continues to grow until puberty, when it begins to atrophy but continues to function. Although its full import is unknown, the thymus produces **T cells** that destroy invading microbes and is thus important to the body's immune system. The ultimobranchial body fuses with the thyroid and contributes parafollicular cells to this gland. Its function is unknown (Figure 3.5).

Vascular Development

Each of the five branchial arches contains a right and a left **aortic arch vessel** that leads from the heart to ascend dorsally through each arch to the face, brain, and posterior regions of the body (see Figure 3.4). Not all of these paired aortic arches are present at the same time, however. The first and second begin to develop in the fourth week and disappear in the fifth week (Figure 3.6). The third arch vessel then becomes prominent and takes over the facial area of the first two. The fourth and fifth arch vessels arise; the fourth remains and the fifth disappears (Figure 3.7). The sixth arises next and becomes, along with the third and fourth vessels, permanent as development continues.

The third arch vessels are the **common carotid arteries** that supply the neck, face, and brain. The fourth arch vessel becomes the **dorsal aorta,** which supplies blood to the entire body, and the vessels of the sixth arch supply the lungs as the **pulmonary circulation** (Figure 3.7).

An interesting feature of these vessels is that the blood supply for the neck and face is first from the internal carotid artery, a branch of the common carotid (Figure 3.8A), but at seven weeks the facial blood supply shifts to the external carotid (Figure 3.8B). The facial vessels detach from the internal carotid and attach to the external carotid, as can be noted in Figure 3.8B. The internal carotid then supplies the enlarging brain.

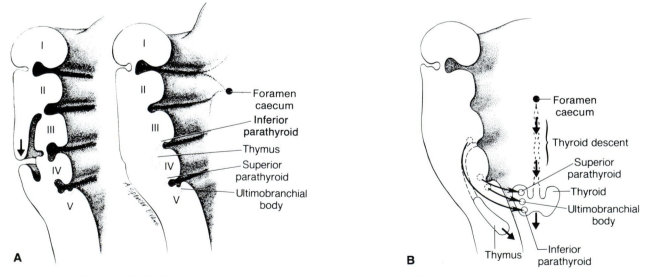

Figure 3.5   **A,** *Overgrowth and disappearance of branchial arches.* **B,** *Contributions of each of pharyngeal pouches.*

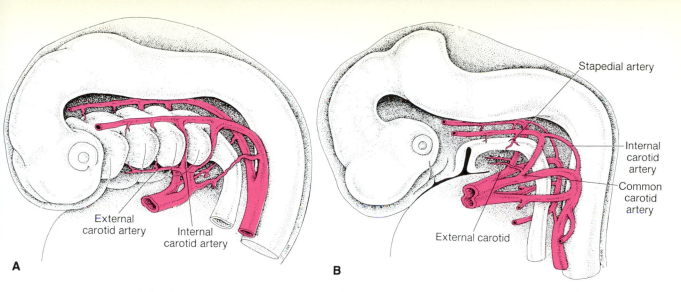

Figure 3.6 *Aortic vasculature development.* **A,** *At 4 weeks the aortic vessels pass through each branchial arch with the pouches between, and then the number 1 and 2 vessels disappear.* **B,** *At 5 weeks the number 3 vessel becomes the common carotid supplying the face by means of the stapedial artery and the brain.*

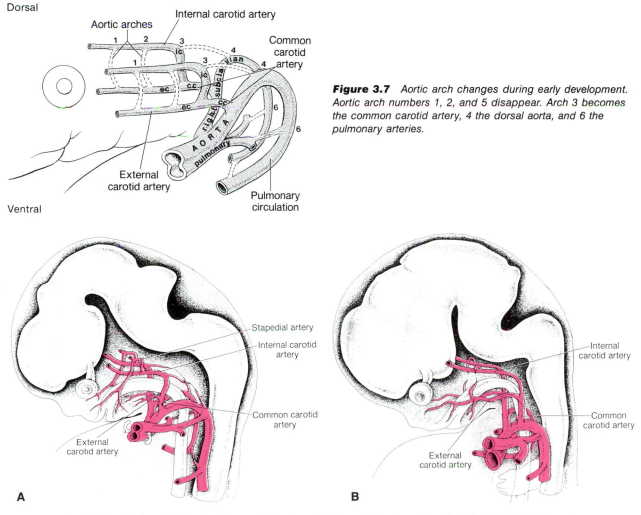

Figure 3.7 *Aortic arch changes during early development. Aortic arch numbers 1, 2, and 5 disappear. Arch 3 becomes the common carotid artery, 4 the dorsal aorta, and 6 the pulmonary arteries.*

Figure 3.8 *Shift in the vascular supply to face.* **A,** *Face and brain are supplied first by the internal carotid artery.* **B,** *There is a loss of attachment of facial vessels to internal carotid artery and attachment to external carotid artery.*

Muscular and Neural Development

Muscle cells in the first arch become apparent during the fifth week and begin to spread within the mandibular arch to each muscle site's origin in the sixth and seventh weeks (Figure 3.9). By the tenth week, the muscles of the second arch have formed a thin sheet that extends over the face and posterior to the ear (Figure 3.10). As these muscles grow over the face, they develop into the various groups of muscles that attach to the newly ossifying bones of the facial skeleton. The muscle masses of the mandibular arch, on the other hand, remain in the first arch and become well organized into recognizable muscles of mastication (see Figure 3.9*A*). These are the **masseter, medial and lateral pterygoid,** and **temporalis muscles.** They all relate to the developing mandible (Figure 3.11).

The masseter and medial pterygoid form a vertical sling inserting into the angle of the mandible. The temporalis muscle spreads into the infratemporal fossa inserting into the developing coronoid process of the mandible. The lateral pterygoid muscle extends horizontally from the neck of the condyle, and some fibers insert into the temporomandibular disc (see Chapter 13). The pharyngeal constrictor muscles in the fourth arch have differentiated in the neck and function to enclose the pharynx (Figure 3.11).

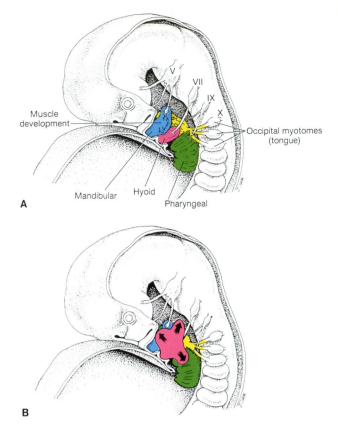

Figure 3.9 *Development of muscles and nerves of branchial arches.* **A,** *Mandibular arch muscle mass expands to form the muscles of mastication.* **B,** *At 7 weeks the muscles of the second arch grow upward to form muscles of face.*

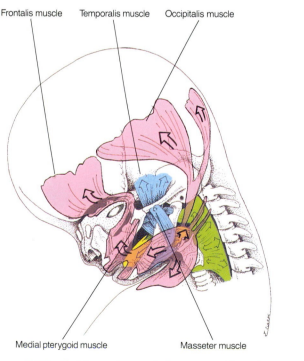

Figure 3.10 *Facial muscle growth from second branchial arch covering the face and scalp and posterior to the ear. These all become the muscles of facial expression.*

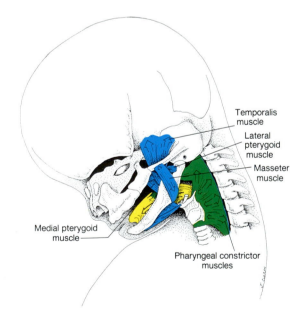

Figure 3.11 *Masticatory muscles of mandibular arch. Observe how medial pterygoid and masseter attach as a sling to the angle of the mandible. Temporalis muscle grows from coronoid process into infratemporal fossa, and lateral pterygoid extends from head of condyle anteriorly to sphenoid and pterygoid bone in infratemporal fossa.*

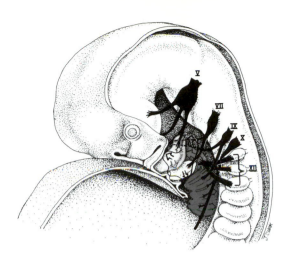

Figure 3.12 *Cranial nerves growing into branchial arches—nerve V to the mandibular arch, nerve VII to the hyoid arch. Nerves IV, VII, IX, and X contribute to anterior developing tongue muscles.*

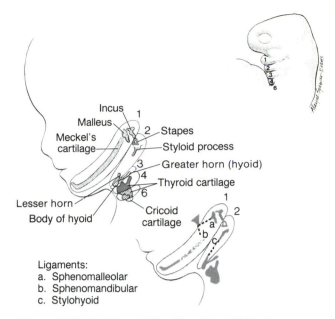

Ligaments:
a. Sphenomalleolar
b. Sphenomandibular
c. Stylohyoid

Figure 3.13 *Cartilage derived from branchial arches—Meckel's cartilage and incus from arch 1; stapes, styloid, and lesser hyoid from arch 2; greater hyoid from arch 3; and thyroid and laryngeal cartilages from arches 4 and 5.*

Nerves develop in conjunction with the muscle fibers. By the seventh week, the fibers of the fifth nerve have entered the mandibular muscle mass as has the seventh nerve in the facial muscle mass in the second arch (Figure 3.12). As these muscle masses develop, the nerves are present and follow and/or lead these muscles as they migrate to their position of function and differentiate. The seventh nerve supplies the stylohyoid and stapedius muscles and the posterior belly of the digastric muscle. The ninth, or glossopharyngeal, nerve enters the third arch and supplies the stylopharyngeal and upper pharyngeal constrictor muscles. The tenth, or vagus, nerve innervates muscles of the fourth arch, which are the inferior constrictors and laryngeal muscles. The tongue muscles relate to the branches of the ninth nerve, which are the receptors of taste for the posterior third of the tongue, and the seventh nerve is the taste receptor of the anterior third or body of the tongue. The fifth serves as the sensory nerve to the same area of the anterior tongue (Figure 3.12).

Cartilaginous Skeletal Development

The initial skeleton of the branchial arches develops as cartilaginous bars. In the first arch, Meckel's cartilages appear bilaterally (Figure 3.13). The anterior cartilage limits approach near the midline but does not fuse with the opposing cartilage. At its posterior limits, Meckel's cartilage terminates in an enlargement, the **malleus,** which is adjacent to but not attached to a small cartilage known as the **incus.** Farther posterior is a third small body of cartilage, **the stapes** (Figure 3.13). These three cartilages later transform into bone and function in the middle ear as hearing bones.

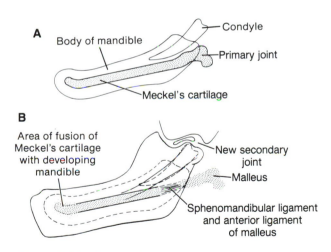

Figure 3.14 *Relationship between primary and secondary jaws. A, Meckel's cartilage with its posterior malleus-incus joint functions in jaw movement during first 4 months of prenatal life. B, There is a shift to the condylar-temporal articulation. Incus and malleus then transform into bones for hearing.*

There is good evidence that the contact point of the malleus and incus is an articulation of the lower jaw for the first 15 to 20 weeks of prenatal life until the second temporomandibular joint, which is the articulation of the condyle and the temporal fossa, becomes functional (Figure 3.14); see Chapter 13.

The rod-shaped cartilage of the second or hyoid arch is known as Reichert's cartilage. The stapes, styloid process, lesser horn and upper part of the body of the hyoid arise from this arch (see Figure 3.13). The third arch cartilage forms the greater horn and the lower part of the hyoid body. The fourth arch contributes to the thyroid cartilage, which then supports this gland. The fifth arch has no adult cartilage derivatives, and the sixth arch cartilage forms the laryngeal cartilages (see Figure 3.13).

■ Development of the Craniofacial Skeleton

Cartilages of the Face

The earliest formed skeletal elements in the craniofacial area are the cartilaginous **nasal (ethmoid) capsule,** the **sphenoid,** the **auditory capsules,** and the **basioccipital cartilages.** All of these cartilages initially arise as a single cartilaginous continuum in the midline underlying the brain (Figure 3.15). Anteriorly, the nasal capsule contains the organ of smell. Laterally, the auditory capsules protect the organs of hearing (Figure 3.15). The sphenoid cartilage is posterior to the ethmoid. It later forms wings of bone that spread out under the developing brain laterally (Figure 3.16). Behind the sphenoid is the occipital cartilage. Although the ethmoid capsule, sphenoid, and basioccipital cartilages are formed as a single cartilaginous unit initially, they separate later to form individual bones. These cartilages underlie and support the brain and are known as the cranial base. The cranial base is determined by drawing a line from the landmarks: the nasal bone, **nasion,** to **sella turcica** of the sphenoid to **basion** as seen in Figure 3.17. These cartilages are transformed into bone by endochondral bone formation.

Bones of the Face

The protective covering of the brain is formed by membrane bones. These bones are termed **frontal, parietal,** and **squamous** portions of the **temporal** and **interoccipital** bones (Figure 3.18). Membrane bones form directly from connective tissue and do not initially form from cartilage, as did the ethmoid and sphenoid bones.

■ Clinical Comment

Branchial arch syndromes are seen clinically as combinations of such defects as underdevelopment of the mandible, retracted tongue, large tongue, small mouth, malformed ears, and cleft palate. A rare disorder, Treacher Collins syndrome, is directly attributable to branchial arch deficiencies.

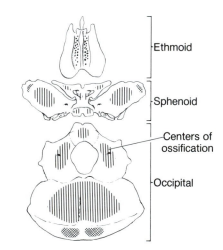

Figure 3.16 *Development of cranial base as viewed in inferior surface of brain. Initiating cartilage centers are shown in center of each site, with bony growth extending outward.*

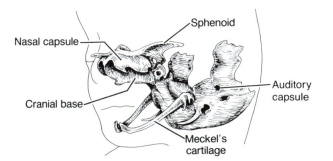

Figure 3.15 *Cartilaginous cartilages of face and skull. Note nasal capsule supporting maxillary area and Meckel's cartilage in the mandibular arch.*

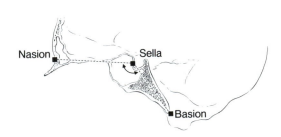

Figure 3.17 *Lateral view of cranial base. A line from nasion to sella to basion is cranial base landmark used to evaluate facial growth.*

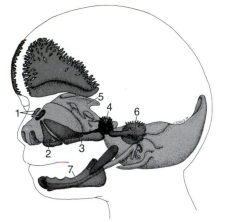

Figure 3.18 *Relationship of cartilage to membrane bony growth of the lateral face at 8 weeks. The facial bones are numbered: 1, Nasal, 2, Premaxilla, 3, Maxilla, 4, Zygomatic, 5, Sphnoid, 6, Temporal, 7, Mandible.*

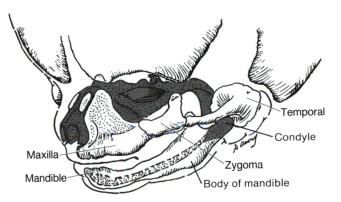

Figure 3.19 *The facial skeleton at the 12th prenatal week illustrating the positional relationships of the maxillary, zygomatic, and temporal bones, and the membrane bone of the body and cartilaginous condyle of the mandible.*

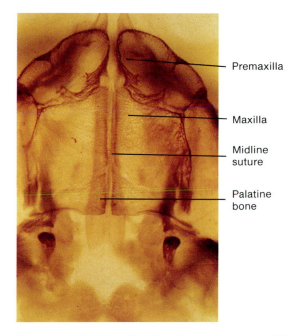

Figure 3.20 *Cleared human specimen. Ossification of human palate in eighth prenatal month. Observe sutures in midline and between each of these bones anteroposteriorly. These provide for further growth of palate. Note developing teeth enclosed in premaxillary, maxillary, and palatine bones.*

The facial bones, which also form in membrane bone, complete the facial skeleton. They develop overlying the nasal capsule and are called the **premaxillary, maxillary, zygomatic,** and **petrous portions** of the **temporal bone** (Figure 3.18). These bones initially appear as tiny ossification centers in the face and then increase in diameter, spreading anteriorly, posteriorly, and upward into the tissues surrounding the orbit (Figure 3.19).

The maxillary bones also grow medially into the palate to support the palatine shelf tissue (Figure 3.20). The bony mandible grows lateral to the first arch cartilage as well as posteriorly to join the bony body with the cartilaginous condyle. Together, the body of the mandible and the cartilaginous condyle replace Meckel's cartilage (see Figure 3.19).

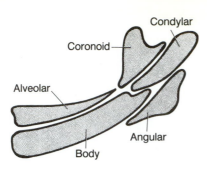

Figure 3.21 *Developing areas of mandible that respond to different influences. The body, condyle, alveolar process, and angular and coronoid processes then all unify as the mandible in common function.*

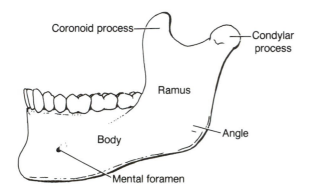

Figure 3.22 *Adult mandibular bone.*

The mandible develops as several units: a **condylar** unit forms the articulation; the **body** is the center of all growth of the mandible; the **angular** unit forms in response to the lateral pterygoid and masseter muscles, the **coronoid** responds to temporalis muscle development; and the **alveolar** unit or process forms in response to the teeth (Figure 3.21). This development produces the mature mandible (Figure 3.22). The bones of the upper face increase in height when the tooth roots begin to form and elongate.

■ *Clinical Comment*

Many facial defects are due to the lack of transformation of the branchial arches into their adult derivatives. Branchial cysts and fistulas may appear along the sides of the neck because the epithelial-lined pockets fail to disappear as a result of the overgrowth of the arches. These defects may also open into the pharynx. These cysts and fistulas may result in swelling or draining of mucus from an opening on the side of the neck.

Sutures of the Face

With further growth of facial bones, a system of articulations is soon required between each of these bones to facilitate future growth. Thus a suture system is formed between the zygomatic, maxillary, frontal and temporal bones, which are separated by the zygomaticomaxillary, zygomaticotemporal, and frontomaxillary sutures (Figure 3.23).

These articulations are defined as growth sites between bones that allow bones to grow and expand and to maintain orientation at their junctions by means of fibrous attachment that controls their relationship with the adjacent bone. Such articulations may consist of a band of connective tissue between bones or they may be composed of cartilage. Connective tissue junctions are characteristic between the facial bones (Figure 3.24), whereas those in the midface are cartilage plates (Figure 3.25). These sutures are called **synchondrosis;** they grow by forming new cartilage at the center of the suture and change into bone along the boundaries of the suture. These cartilage junctions are of only one type; connective tissue articulations termed **syndesmosis** which are of three types: **simple,** positioned at the interface of adjacent bones (Figure 3.24); **serrated,** an interdigitating type of suture (Figure 3.26); and **squamosal** (squamous suture), an overlapping or beveled suture (Figure 3.27). These names are descriptive, as evident when one examines any of these sutures.

The sutures expand through growth of connective tissue and bone. Each suture consists of a central zone of proliferating connective tissue cells, with osteogenic cells along the peripheral bony fronts, which are surrounded by fibrous connective tissue (see Figures 3.24 to 3.27). When the position of the sutures in the fetal skull is compared with that in the adult skull, it can be seen that the relationships of these articulations are similar, although the adult bones are larger (Figure 3.28).

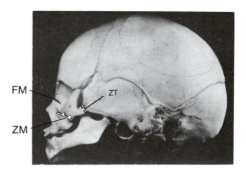

Figure 3.23 *Sutures of developing skull of the newborn human. FM = frontomaxillary; ZM = zygomaticomaxillary; ZT = zygomaticotemporal. The pterygopalatine suture is not shown; note its position in Figure 3.28.*

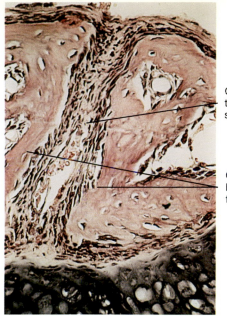

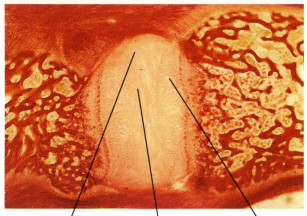

Resting zone   Proliferative zone   Ossification zone

Figure 3.25 *Histology of synchondrosis. This band of cartilage develops by growth of new cartilage in center of this suture and cartilage replacement by bone peripherally along the bony fronts.*

Connective tissue of suture

Opposing bone fronts

Figure 3.24 *Histology of simple suture illustrating opposing bone fronts above and below with connective tissue between. Osteoblasts form bone on opposing bone fronts, causing growth, and connective tissue band maintains space between them, allowing more osteoblasts to develop.*

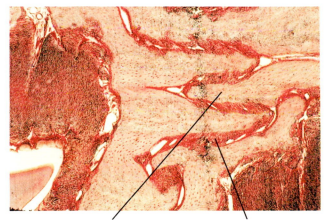

Interdigitating bone   Connective tissue of suture

Figure 3.26 *Histology of serrated suture of skull. Observe interposing (interdigitating) fingers of bone with connective tissue between each of these projections.*

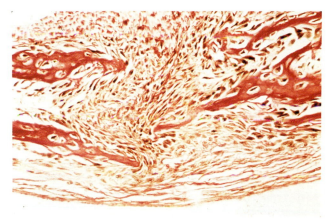

Figure 3.27 *Histology of squamous suture of skull. The bones of suture overlap and have connective tissue between.*

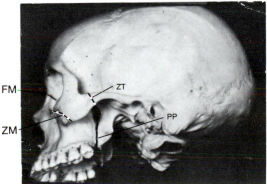

Figure 3.28 *Sutures of the adult human skull. FM = frontomaxillary; ZM = zygomaticomaxillary; ZT zygomaticotemporal; PP = pterygopalatine. Compare their position with that of the newborn in Figure 3.23.*

■ *Self-Evaluation Questions*

1. Define a branchial arch.
2. Describe the origin of the facial muscles.
3. Enumerate several important events that take place in the second branchial arch between the fourth and seventh weeks of gestation.
4. Discuss the shift of the blood supply from the internal to the external carotid vessels.
5. What are the contributions of the first branchial groove and pharyngeal pouch?
6. Describe the path of descent of the thyroid gland.
7. What are the origin and function of the parathyroid glands?
8. What cartilaginous skeleton is found in each of the arches?
9. Name and locate the sutures of the face.
10. Name and locate the cartilages of the cranial base.

■ *Suggested Reading*

Enlow, D.H. Handbook of facial growth. Philadelphia: W.B. Saunders, 1982.

Hall, B.K. Development and skeletal biology. New York: Academic Press, 1978.

Sadler, T. Langman's medical embryology, 5th ed. Baltimore: Williams & Wilkins, 1985.

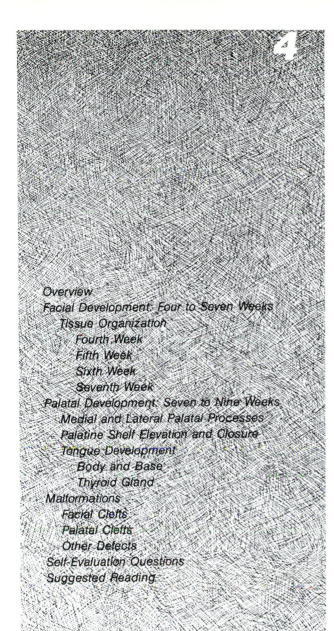

Development of the Face and the Palate

■ Overview

The development of the human face and palate and defects that may occur are described in this chapter. An understanding of this subject is important to the dental health professional for two reasons. One first must understand the variability that can occur in facial form, and, second, must have an awareness that the human face and palate are among the areas most susceptible to malformations.

The human face develops early in gestation, during the fifth through seventh weeks, and the palatal processes begin to close during the eighth week. These two structures are closely related in time of development and may have related malformations. The face develops from those tissues immediately surrounding the oral pit, but the forehead develops from the frontal area that lies above the pit (see Figure 4.1). Later, the nose develops from this area as well, so the name changes from frontal area to frontonasal area (see Figure 4.2). Below the oral pit is the mandibular arch, from which the mandible arises and articulates with the temporal bone. Lateral to the oral pit are the right and left maxillary processes, which develop from the mandibular arch. These processes give rise to the tissues of the cheeks.

Intraorally, the palate forms the roof of the mouth, which separates the oral and nasal cavities. First, the medial palatal segment forms, which is a part of the medial nasal lip segment. This segment provides the first separation of the oral and nasal cavities. Next, two lateral palatine shelves arise from the maxillary processes, which then grow horizontally to close the palate posterior to the pharynx. The tongue first develops in the floor of the oral cavity but grows rapidly to expand into the nasal cavity. It plays a role in palatine shelf closure because the shelves must first override the tongue before palatal closure can be accomplished.

Many environmental factors can cause cleft of the face, palate, or both. These defects of the lip or palate may be unilateral or bilateral and incomplete or complete.

■ *Facial Development: Four to Seven Weeks*

Tissue Organization

The face develops primarily from those tissues surrounding the oral pit. Above the oral area is the covering of the brain termed the **frontal process** from which develops the forehead. Lateral to the oral pit are two **maxillary processes,** which form the cheeks, and below is the **mandibular arch,** which forms the lower jaw. In the fourth week, when the facial tissues are organizing, they measure a few millimeters in width and height and are as thick as a sheet of paper. Further growth of the face, from this assembly of minute tissue sites, is anterior from the brain. The second branchial or **hyoid arch** lies inferior to the mandibular arch, and its muscles extend into and contribute to the face. The hyoid arch also forms part of the external and middle ear.

Development of the human face is most easily described in terms of the changes that occur at weekly intervals, from the fourth to seventh prenatal weeks.

Fourth Week

At four weeks, the oral pit is seen with several masses of tissue surrounding it, and several branchial arches are evident below it and on the sides of the neck. The frontal processes of the brain bulge forward and laterally to dominate the facial area. Below the frontal processes are two small wedge-shaped tissues that lie lateral to the pit termed the maxillary process. Beneath the maxillary process is the mandibular arch, which appears divided or constricted in the midline (Figure 4.1). The bulging heart below the mandible lies in the thorax, but it must be removed to allow visualization of the area during the fourth week.

Fifth Week

During the fifth week, bilateral **nasal placodes,** or thickened areas of epithelium, appear on the upper border of the lip. They develop into nostrils as the tissues around these placodes grow, resulting in two slits opening into the oral pit. At this point, the frontal area becomes known as the frontonasal process. In the fifth week, the nostrils deepen as the tissues around the nostrils continue to grow, and the internasal area, the distance between the nostrils, represents most of the width of the face (Figure 4.2). The tissues lateral to the nostrils are termed the lateral nasal, and the tissue medial to the nostrils is called the medial nasal process. Gradually, the frontal prominences diminish and the face broadens. The eyes become prominent on the sides of the head during the fifth week (see Figure 4.2).

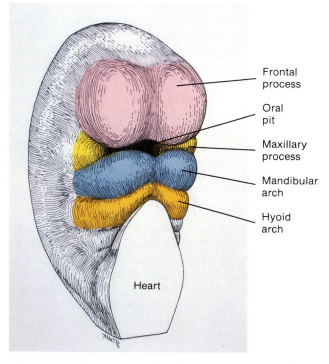

Figure 4.1 *Human face during the fourth prenatal week. Frontal and maxillary processes and mandibular arch, though seemingly unrelated tissue masses, are grouped around oral pit. Below mandibular arch is hyoid arch. Heart is also shown below face.*

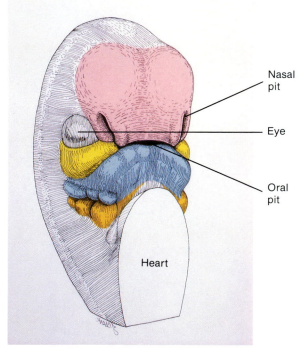

Figure 4.2 *Human face during the fifth prenatal week. Nasal pits are located laterally in face during this week. Frontal process changes to the frontonasal process.*

Sixth Week

At the beginning of the sixth week, the lateral parts of the face expand, broadening the face. This causes the location of the eyes to change from the side of the head to the front. The oral pit then widens to become a slit that extends laterally to merge with each maxillary process and the mandibular arch. The upper lip is composed of two lateral maxillary segments and a medial nasal part. The medial nasal process (Figure 4.3) is also called the **philtrum.** A ridge of tissue surrounds each nasal pit. The tissue lateral to the pits is the lateral nasal process, and that medial to it is the nasal process. The medial nasal process contacts each maxillary process to effect lip closure. These three parts of the lip then fuse, unifying the lip (Figure 4.3). A lack of contact or fusion at these points will result in a cleft lip, either unilateral or bilateral. The epithelial covering of the medial nasal and maxillary processes forms a zone of contact called the **nasal fin** (Figure 4.4). This epithelial fin is soon penetrated by connective tissue growth, which binds the parts of the lip (Figure 4.4). If this does not occur, the lip can pull apart. Later, the **orbicularis oris muscle** grows around the lip to provide support. Extending from the nostrils to the eye is an oblique groove. Deep beneath this groove the **nasolacrimal duct** develops. At this time, the mandibular arch broadens and loses the midline constriction (see Figure 4.3). There also appears a modification of the first branchial groove into an ear canal, or **auditory tube,** below the corners of the mouth. Six small hillocks of tissue are grouped around this external ear canal. Three of these are contributed by the mandibular arch and three from the hyoid arch (see Figures 4.3 and 4.6).

■ Clinical Comment

Environmental factors play a significant role in facial and palatal malformations. The period prior to the fifth week is the critical time during which these factors can affect facial development.

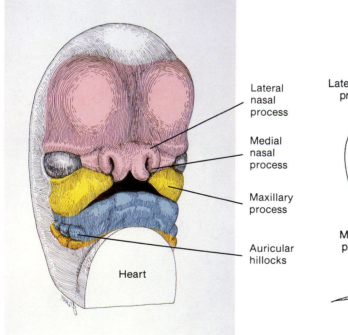

Figure 4.3 *Human face during the sixth prenatal week. Nasal pits appear more centrally located in medial nasal process. Growth in lateral area of face causes eyes to approach front of face. Nasal slits may be sites of cleft lips. Hillocks of ear have merged.*

Lateral nasal process

Medial nasal process

Maxillary process

Auricular hillocks

Heart

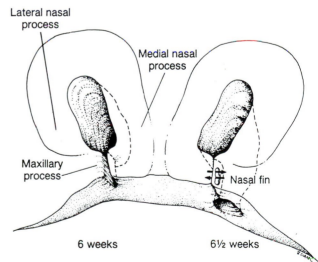

Lateral nasal process

Medial nasal process

Maxillary process

Nasal fin

6 weeks

6½ weeks

Figure 4.4 *Fusion of floor of the nostrils. Observe at left, the epithelial covering of the medial nasal and maxillary processes. At right, the processes are in contact and fused, and the epithelial layers then form a fin. This fin is later penetrated by connective tissue, which grows through the epithelium to bind the lip crevice.*

Seventh Week

By the seventh week the face has begun to take on a more human appearance (Figure 4.5). As the eyes approach the front of the face, the nose represents less of the face than it did just a few days previously. The lateral growth of the forebrain causes the eyes to appear on the front of the face and the nostrils to appear more centrally located. This is due to the addition of a third of the face lateral to each nostril (Figure 4.5). The eyes are on the same horizontal plane as the nostrils, which will change later as the bridge of the nose develops and lengthens. The upper lip has fused, producing a medially located philtrum. The mouth is now limited in size with the change in facial proportions. The ear hillocks have fused to form the ears, and the ridges around the eyes will soon develop eyelids (Figures 4.5 and 4.6). In just three weeks, from the fourth to the seventh, a group of separate tissue masses have enlarged, fused, and merged into a recognizable human face.

■ *Clinical Comment*

Because much of the face arises from the tissues lying on the surface of the brain, defects of the anterior brain may result in a developmental alteration of facial form.

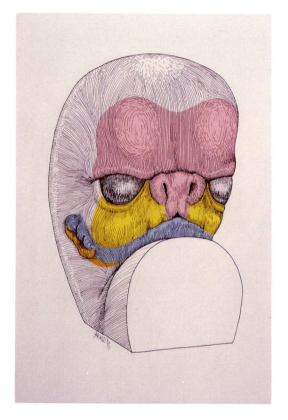

Figure 4.5 *Human face during seventh prenatal week. Median nasal and maxillary processes have merged. Eyes are nearer the front of face. Nose and eyes are on same horizontal plane, which will later change with vertical growth of the face. Auricles of the ears have developed.*

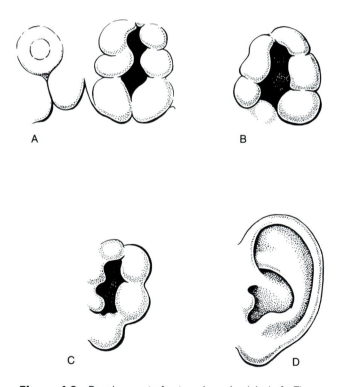

Figure 4.6 *Development of external ear (auricles).* **A,** *The three auricular hillocks on left are from mandibular arch, and three on right are from hyoid arch.* **B,** *Auricular hillocks merge around the first branchial groove.* **C,** *The hillocks merge.* **D,** *The ear is developed.*

■ Palatal Development: Seven to Nine Weeks

Medial and Lateral Palatal Processes

The human palate is that tissue that separates the oral and nasal cavities. This palate, although thin, is supported by bone, which provides rigidity. The palate develops from three parts: an anterior wedge-shaped medial part and two lateral palatine processes (Figure 4.7A). The medial part is also known as the **primary palate,** since it develops as a floor to the nasal pits. Next, the **lateral palatine processes** develop out of the maxillary tissues laterally and grow to the midline. This further limits the oral cavity from the nasal cavity posteriorly to the nasopharynx (Figure 4.7B). The palatine shelves first grow medially until they meet the tongue. The tongue has grown extensively dorsally during the seventh week, until it enters the nasal cavity. When the shelves contact the tongue, they grow downward on either side of the tongue (Figure 4.8).

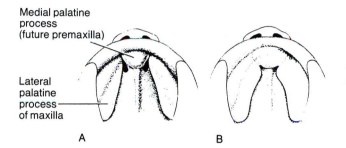

Medial palatine process (future premaxilla)

Lateral palatine process of maxilla

A   B

Figure 4.7 *Development of palate.* **A,** *Early development of medial and lateral palatine processes.* **B,** *Developing lateral palatine processes.*

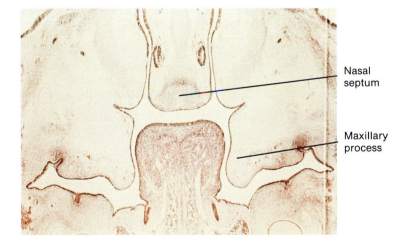

Nasal septum

Maxillary process

Figure 4.8 *Palatine shelves contact tongue and then grow down beside it during seventh week. Tongue muscle differentiates at this time as does cartilage in the nasal area above.*

Palatine Shelf Elevation and Closure

At its posterior limits the tongue is below the palatine shelves. This is because the tongue is attached to the floor of the mouth and the roof of the posterior palate is high. During the eighth week, the posterior shelves push together, forcing the tongue forward (Figure 4.9). Such action allows the shelves to push the tongue forward, and then the shelves slide forward over the tongue (Figure 4.10). This process is known as **palatine shelf elevation** and is presumed to occur rapidly, about as fast as the act of swallowing. For this reason, palatine shelf elevation action has never been precisely recorded. As soon as the palatine shelves have reached the resulting horizontal position, the tongue broadens and lies beneath the shelves (Figure 4.11). There is a final medial growth increase of the shelves, until they contact in the midline, which is known as **palatine shelf closure** (Figure 4.12). As soon as the shelves meet or contact in the midline, **fusion** occurs. The first site of fusion is just posterior to the medial palatine process (Figure 4.12). From this point of initial contact, the two shelves merge in both a posterior and an anterior direction (Figure 4.12). The final step in fusion is the removal of the midline epithelial barrier between the right and left shelves. This occurs through the self-destruction of epithelial cells, as seen in Figure 4.13. The process takes some weeks as the shelves continue to lengthen and widen. These palatine shelves also fuse with the overlying nasal septum in the midline, which causes a complete separation of the nasal cavities from the oral cavity posterior to the oropharynx (Figure 4.13).

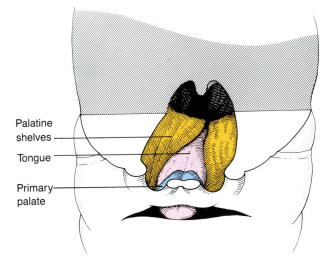

Figure 4.9 *Palatine shelves position beside tongue anteriorly and above it posteriorly.*

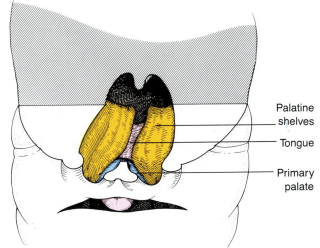

Figure 4.10 *Palatine shelf elevation over tongue. Observe tongue's position as palatine shelves move it anteriorly during their elevation process.*

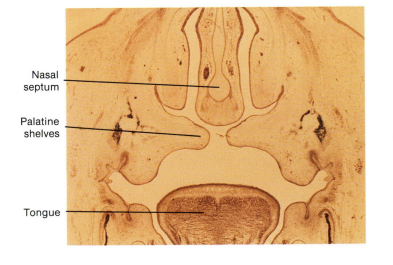

Figure 4.11 *Cross section of tongue beneath palatine shelves. Shelves are in near median contact as well as contact above with nasal septum.*

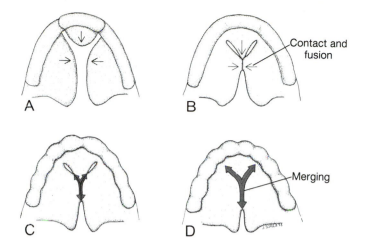

Figure 4.12 **A,** *Horizontal palatine shelf growth to attain contact in the midline.* **B,** *Initial contact behind medial palatal segment.* **C,** *and* **D,** *Tissue merges anteriorly and posteriorly from that point.*

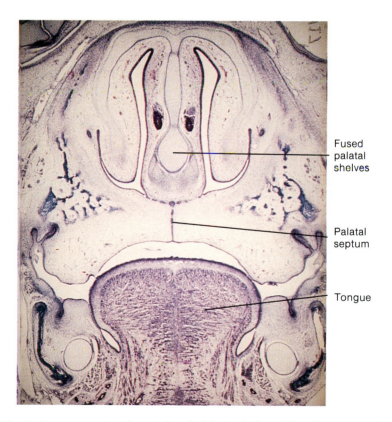

Figure 4.13 *Histologic cross section of a palatine shelf fusion in the midline. On contact, the epithelial seam breaks down between the shelves and with overlying septum.*

Tongue Development

Body and Base

The tongue originates from the muscles of the occipital somites (see Figures 3.9 to 3.11). From this posterior location, the forming muscles migrate anteriorly into the floor of the mouth and are joined by other muscles of the first and second branchial arches. The tongue is innervated by the fifth, seventh, ninth, and tenth cranial nerves. This large number of nerves is due to their migration forward along with the occipital muscle groups (see Chapter 3). The first arch tissue forms the anterior movable part, the body of the tongue; the second and third arches form the posterior less movable tongue base. Tissues of the tongue body are composed of three parts, the central **tuberculum impar** and the two **lateral lingual swellings** (Figure 4.14). These lateral parts rapidly enlarge and merge with each other, overgrowing the central tubercle. A U-shaped sulcus then develops around the anterior part of the tongue, separating it from the jaw tissues, which allows freedom of movement (Figure 4.15). Gradually, the three parts of the anterior tongue merge to form a unified structure. The surface of the body and base of the tongue are separated by a V-shaped groove, called the **terminal sulcus.** Posterior to this, the base of the tongue forms the **lingual tonsil** on its dorsal surface. This forms part of the ring of tonsils along with the **palatine** and **pharyngeal tonsils** that form in the pharynx. In later stages of development, several types of papillae differentiate on the dorsal mucosa of the tongue's body, and the lymphatic tonsil differentiates on the surface of the tongue's base.

Thyroid Gland

The thyroid gland develops as an epithelial proliferation from the foramen on the surface of the tongue in the midline of the terminal sulcus. In the center of this sulcus, there is an opening where cells arise and migrate ventrally in the throat to give rise to the thyroid gland (Figure 4.15). This opening, termed the **foramen caecum,** is the site of the thyroid tissue. It then descends in the midline floor of the pharynx past the hyoid cartilages to the level of the laryngeal cartilages, and finally, by the seventh week, it goes to the front of the trachea. During this migration, the gland remains attached to the tongue by an epithelial cord or duct termed the **thyroglossal duct** (see Figure 3.5*B*). This duct then becomes solid and eventually disappears (Figure 4.16).

Cysts and fistulas can be found along the route of descent of the thyroid tissue. A **thyroglossal cyst** is a blind pocket lined with thyroid epithelium. This cyst appears as a swelling and is commonly found in the area of the hyoid bone. A thyroglossal fistula appears as a swelling that has an opening on the surface of the neck (Figure 4.17).

The gland finally acquires two lateral lobes joined by a thin central isthmus of cells. By the end of the third month of prenatal life, the gland becomes functional.

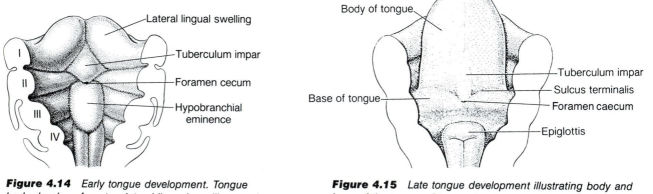

Figure 4.14 *Early tongue development. Tongue body develops from two lateral lingual swellings and a midline tuberculum impar. Tongue base develops from second and third branchial arches.*

Figure 4.15 *Late tongue development illustrating body and base of the tongue. Observe location of foramen caecum, which is site of origin of tubular epithelial cord growth down the neck, which gives rise to the thyroid gland.*

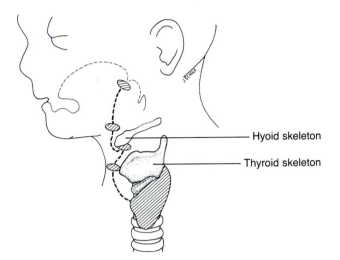

Hyoid skeleton

Thyroid skeleton

Figure 4.16 *Migratory path of thyroid gland tissue. Sometimes epithelial cysts and fistulas arise along this path of descent. Site may be in region of the thyro-hyoid skeleton.*

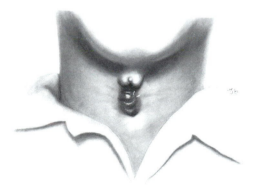

Figure 4.17 *Clinical view of thyroglossal duct fistula appearing at midline of neck, in region of hyoid apparatus. This is usual location.*

■ *Malformations*

Facial and palatal clefts usually occur because of a combination of environmental and genetic factors. This fact leads to consideration of the individual's susceptibility to stress, which can produce adverse effects.

Cleft lip is the most common facial malformation. Genetic factors play a role, as shown by the fact that among the white American population the incidence of cleft lip is 1 in every 700 births. A greater number, more than 3 in 2,000, occur in the Asian population. Asians with one child born with a cleft palate have a 1 in 25 chance of having a second child with the defect. Proportionately, there are significantly fewer black Americans who are affected with clefts, the incidence being only 1 in 2,000 newborns. This disparity is not surprising, since any congenital malformation affects each race at a different ratio from the others. Evidence clearly shows that a predominant hereditary role exists along with various environmental susceptibility factors. The incidence of clefts in males and females are also different.

White males have, proportionately, nearly twice the number of cleft lips or cleft lips and palates as females. However, more white females than males have cleft palates which occur in about 1 in every 2,000 live births. Overall, though, cleft palate is less frequent than cleft lip or combination of cleft lip and palate.

Facial Clefts

Facial clefts are classified according to position and extent of injury. A cleft may affect one or both sides of the lip and can be either incomplete or complete (unilateral or bilateral) (Figures 4.18 to 4.20). The incomplete cleft lip may range in size from a notch to a deep groove in the lip but does not involve an opening of the nostril into the oral cavity (Figure 4.18). A true harelip is a midline cleft of the maxilla. The term harelip is used because the upper lip of the rabbit develops with a midline cleft. The condition, which is rare in humans, involves a notch in the medial nasal tissue that may be minute or extend as a cleft into the nose (Figure

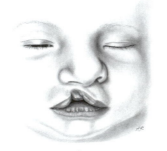

Figure 4.18 *Clinical view of unilateral incomplete cleft of the lip. This partial cleft is located in line of fusion of medial nasal and maxillary processes.*

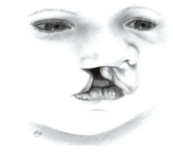

Figure 4.19 *Clinical view of unilateral complete cleft of the lip. In this case, the two processes failed to fuse and then pulled farther apart as development continued.*

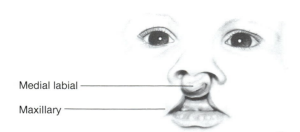

Medial labial

Maxillary

Figure 4.20 *Clinical view of bilateral complete cleft of the lip. Maxillary and medial labial and palatal tissues then extrude anteriorly.*

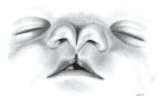

Figure 4.21 *Clinical view of midline cleft of the maxilla. This rare cleft occurs when the two parts of the medial nasal process fail to merge.*

4.21). A cleft of the mandible may appear in the midline, although this also is rare (Figure 4.22). The midline constriction in Figure 4.1 was seen in the fourth week. In this case, the early constriction did not disappear but continued and later resulted in a separation. This is believed due to pressure of the adjacent enlarging heart that begins beating in the fourth week.

Palatal Clefts

All the preceding facial clefts are those of the lip only, but these may extend into the palate as unilateral or bilateral cleft lip and palate defects as well (Figure 4.23). Because the palatine shelves meet in the midline, both unilateral and bilateral clefts of the palate are midline clefts. Clefts must, however, extend around the medial palatal segment before proceeding into the midline (Figure 4.23). Just as clefts of the lip can occur alone, the clefts of the palate may occur as

an isolated defect (Figure 4.23*B*). These palatal clefts may extend just a short distance into the posterior of the palate or may appear in the anterior plate, or they may appear in both locations. However, the majority of cleft palates occur in combination with cleft lips (Figures 4.24 and 4.25).

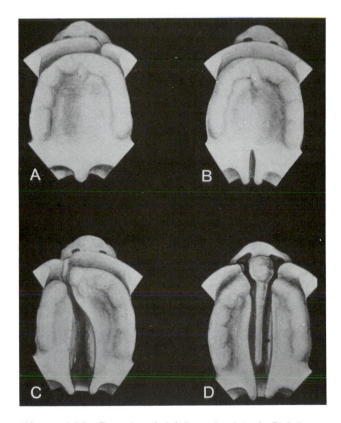

Figure 4.23 *Examples of cleft lip and palate.* **A,** *Cleft lip alone.* **B,** *Cleft of palate alone.* **C,** *Unilateral cleft lip and palate.* **D,** *Bilateral cleft lip and palate.*

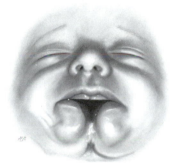

Figure 4.22 *Clinical example of midline cleft of the mandible. In this rare defect, the two parts of the first branchial arch are separated in the midline.*

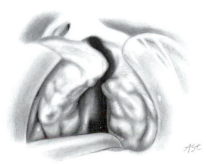

Figure 4.24 *Combined unilateral cleft of palate and lip. Observe how these clefts go lateral to the medial palatal segment and then posteriorly in the midline between the two palatine processes. Observe distortion of nasal tissue.*

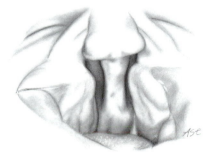

Figure 4.25 *Combined bilateral cleft of palate and lip. Observe cleft extending lateral to medial process and then down midline.*

Other Defects

A number of other facial deformities are seen clinically, some of which are common and others very rare. The origin of, for example, an oronasal optic cleft, a cleft extending from the mouth to the eye, can be seen in Figure 4.3. The most common defects are various malocclusions of the teeth. Midfacial hypoplasia—for example, Crouzon's and Apert's disease—is a less common abnormality. The developmental aspects of the first and second branchial arch syndromes were described in Chapter 3.

■ *Clinical Comment*

Cleft lip and palate are one of the more common congenital malformations. They appear in 1 of every 700 births in the white population and 1 in 2,000 in the black population in the United States.

■ *Self-Evaluation Questions*

1. From what four processes does the face arise?
2. During which three prenatal weeks does the human face develop? When does the face take on a human appearance?
3. When do the palatine shelves elevate and begin closure?
4. The upper lip is composed of three segments: name them. When do they coalesce into one unit?
5. From what structure does the nasal fin arise, and why is its disappearance important?
6. From what tissue do the external ears develop?
7. Define the primary and secondary palates, and explain when each appears and their relative importance.
8. Describe the process of palatine shelf elevation.
9. From what three tissue masses does the tongue form?
10. Compare the ratios of facial and palatal defects in the white, Asian, and black American populations.

■ *Suggested Reading*

Moore, K.L. Human embryology. Toronto: B.C. Decker, 1988.

Sadler, T., ed. Langman's medical embryology, 5th ed. Baltimore: Williams & Wilkins, 1985.

Snyder, G.B., Berkowitz, S., Bzoch, K.R., and Stool, S. Your cleft lip and palate child. Gainesville, Fla.: Florida Cleft Palate Association and Mead Johnson Laboratories, 1972.

Sperber, G.H. Craniofacial embryology, 4th ed. London: Butterworth, 1989.

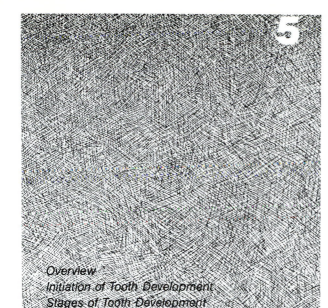

Development of the Teeth

■ Overview

Tooth development results from an interaction of the oral epithelial cells and the underlying mesenchymal cells. From this interaction, 20 primary and 32 permanent teeth develop. Each developing tooth grows as an anatomically distinct unit. The fundamental developmental process is similar for all teeth.

Each tooth develops through successive bud, cap, and bell stages (Figure 5.1A to C). During these early stages, the tooth germs grow and expand, and the cells that are to form the hard tissues of the teeth then differentiate. Once this occurs in the bell stage, the stages of dentinogenesis and amelogenesis take place (Figure 5.1D and E). After the crowns and roots of these teeth form and mineralize, the supporting tissues of the teeth, cementum, periodontal ligament, and alveolar bone begin to form (Figure 5.1F and G). This formation occurs whether the tooth is an incisor with a single root or a molar with multiple roots. Subsequently, the completed tooth crown erupts into the oral cavity (Figure 5.1G). Root formation and cementogenesis then proceed until a functional tooth and its supporting apparatus are fully developed (Figure 5.1G and H).

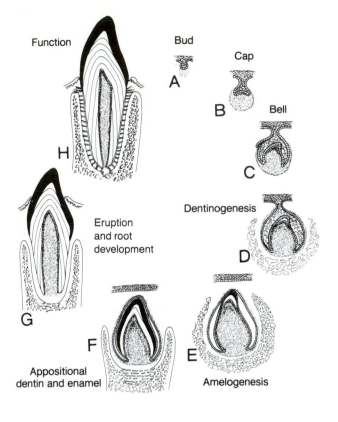

Figure 5.1 (A to H) *The stages of tooth development from the bud stage to function.*

■ Initiation of Tooth Development

Teeth develop from two types of cells—oral epithelial cells that give rise to the enamel organ and mesenchymal cells from which the dental papillae cells arise. Enamel develops from the enamel organ and dentin from the dental papilla. The interaction of these epithelial cells and the mesenchyme is vital to the initiation and formation of the teeth.

Neural crest cells are synonymous with the mesenchymal cells of the head and neck. These cells induce or interact with the epithelial cells to form the teeth and salivary glands. They also function in the formation of bone, cartilage, nerves, and muscles of the face. The role of the neural crest cells is not completely understood, although it is known that they are derived from the cells of the neural folds and then migrate down the sides of the head and into the jaws, where they begin functioning.

In the jaws, the neural crest cells induce the oral epithelium to proliferate and form the **dental lamina,** which is the first sign of tooth development. This lamina then invaginates as a sheet of epithelial cells into the underlying mesenchyme around the perimeter of both the maxillary and mandibular jaws (Figure 5.2). Along the leading edges of the lamina 20 areas of enlargement next appear, which

are the forming buds of the 20 primary teeth (Figure 5.2). These buds then develop into the primary teeth, and the leading edge of the lamina continues to develop the 32 permanent tooth buds (Figure 5.3).

Successional tooth buds form the permanent dentition lingual to the buds of the primary predecessors (see Figure 5.3). The lingual extension of the dental lamina that gives rise to the successional teeth is therefore called the successional lamina (Figure 5.3). Permanent molars develop posterior to the primary molars, and the general dental lamina grows posteriorly to form the permanent molar buds. The last teeth to arise from the dental lamina are the third molars, which develop in about the fifteenth year after birth. Since these teeth do not succeed the primary teeth, they form not from the successional lamina but from the general lamina (Figure 5.3). The dental lamina is thus functional in developing the 52 teeth from the sixth prenatal week until 15 years after birth. Because the primary tooth buds form anteroposteriorly, they are more advanced in the anterior jaws (see Figure 5.2). After the primary teeth have developed and their crowns erupt and become functional, the permanent tooth buds are just beginning to develop. This same process then takes place in the more posterior portion of the jaws, where permanent molar teeth are not succedaneous replacements for the primary teeth.

■ Clinical Comment

Tooth formation is dependent on both oral epithelial and adjacent mesenchymal cells for development. Factors such as x-rays, nutritional deficiencies, and drugs can alter the ability of these cells to function, thus affecting tooth development.

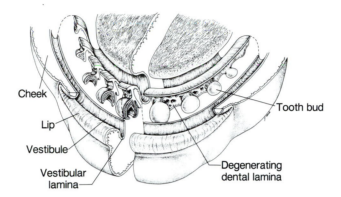

Figure 5.2 *Development of tooth buds in the alveolar process. Note the anterior teeth are more advanced in development over the posterior teeth and the anterior lamina is degenerating.*

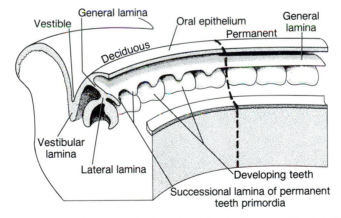

Figure 5.3 *The dental lamina system is shown in relation to the general lamina. The successional lamina gives rise to the permanent teeth, which replace the primary teeth except in the posterior area of the arch.*

■ Stages of Tooth Development

Although tooth formation is a continuous process, it is characterized by a series of easily distinguishable stages known as the bud, cap, and bell stages. They are defined according to the shape of the epithelial enamel organ segment of the developing tooth. The **bud stage,** or first stage, is the rounded localized growth of the epithelial cells of the enamel organ (Figure 5.4*A* and *B*). Gradually the round epithelial bud gains a concave surface, and the enamel organ is then considered to be in the **cap stage** of development (Figure 5.5). The cap stage consists of an enamel organ, dental papilla, and the area around these structures known as the **dental follicle.**

After further increase in size of the enamel organ and adjacent dental papilla, the tooth germ reaches the **bell stage.** At this stage the enamel organ has differentiated ιnto (1) the **outer enamel epithelial** (OEE) cells, which cover the outer convex surface of the enamel organ; (2) the **inner enamel epithelial** (IEE) cells, which first form the outline of the future shape of the tooth crown; (3) a layer of cells adjacent to the inner enamel epithelial cells, which are within the enamel organ and are termed the **stratum inter-**

medium (SI) cells; and (4) those cells that fill the remainder of the enamel organ, which are termed the **stellate reticulum** (SR) cells (Figure 5.6). This is the differentiation stage, and it exhibits two characteristics: (1) the inner enamel epithelial cells define the shape of the future tooth crown to be formed, and (2) the inner enamel epithelial cells elongate and differentiate into **ameloblasts** to become the future enamel-forming cells. Adjacent to the ameloblasts, the layer of stratum intermedium cells appear spindle-shaped and function with the ameloblasts in the formation of the enamel. The epithelial cells of the outer enamel become associated with a capillary plexus, which functions to bring nutrition to the ameloblasts and other enamel organ cells (Figure 5.6). During this bell stage, the cells in the periphery of the dental papilla differentiate into **odontoblasts.** They elongate and function in dentin formation.

The general and lateral dental laminae begin to degenerate at the bell stage. The tooth bud differentiates and becomes independent of the oral epithelium. In this process, the epithelial cells undergo lysis and the dental lamina disappears (see Figure 5.2). The general lamina is maintained more posteriorly in the mouth, however, where other teeth are less advanced in development (see Figure 5.3).

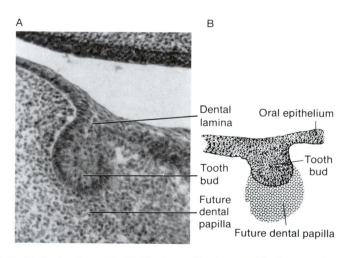

Figure 5.4 *Tooth development: (A) histology of bud stage, (B) diagram of the same.*

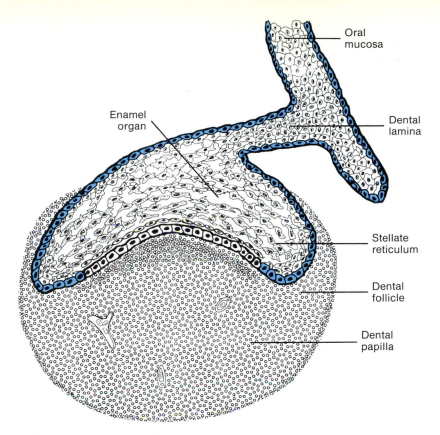

Figure 5.5   *Tooth development. Diagram of cap stage.*

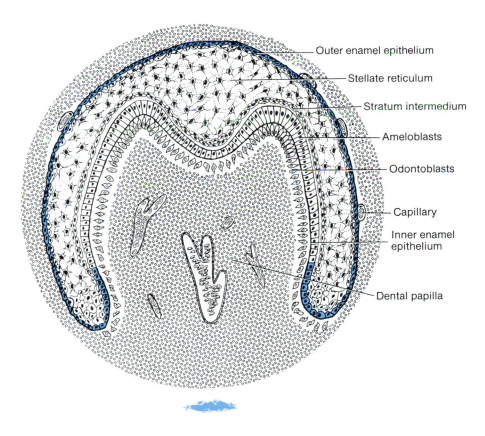

Figure 5.6   *Tooth development. Diagram of bell stage.*

■ Development of the Dental Papilla or Pulp Organ

The young dental papilla is more densely packed with cells than are the tissues surrounding the teeth. In Figure 5.7, two primary maxillary and mandibular molar buds are seen in the jaw. The high cell density of the pulps indicates the increased cell division and growth of the papilla, which will keep pace with the growth of the enamel organ.

On closer examination, the cells of the pulp organ are seen to be fibroblasts and appear in a delicate reticulum (Figure 5.8). A few larger blood vessels traverse the central area of the pulp, and smaller ones are seen in its periphery. Although large nerve trunks are located near the developing young teeth, only a few small nerves associated with blood vessels enter the developing young pulp. Later, as the teeth erupt and come into function, the larger myelinated nerves become more abundant throughout the pulp organ.

The peripheral cells of the dental papilla then transform into columnar-shaped cells and develop cell processes. They are then known as odontoblasts (see Figure 5.6).

In summary, dental papilla cells first induce the epithelial cells of the inner enamel to differentiate. The epithelial cells of the inner enamel then induce the odontoblasts to differentiate and are ready to form dentin before the ameloblasts form enamel (see Figure 5.6).

■ Dentinogenesis

As the odontoblasts begin dentin formation, this process is termed dentinogenesis (Figure 5.8). The dental papilla becomes surrounded by dentin, and it is then termed the dental pulp (Figure 5.8). The pulp organ and dentin are closely related because the dentin-forming odontoblasts reside in the periphery of the pulp, where they form the dentinal matrix. Odontoblasts maintain cell processes within the dentinal tubules. When the odontoblasts move pulpward away from the basal lamina, they deposit collagen fibrils and associated organic matter, as seen in Figures 5.9 and 5.10*A, B,* and *C.*

When odontoblasts start functioning, their nuclei occupy a more basal position in the cell, and the cell organelles become more evident within the cells. The appearance of granular endoplasmic reticulum, Golgi's complex, and mitochondria indicates the protein-producing nature of these cells (Figure 5.10*C* to *E*). The cells then secrete the protein externally via vesicles at the apical part of the cell and along the cell process (Figure 5.10). The collagenous dentinal matrix is not mineralized when it is first deposited and is therefore termed predentin. As this collagen matrix forms, the odontoblasts move farther away from what will become the dentinoenamel junction (DEJ), which can be noted in Figures 5.9 to 5.10. The cell process elongates and resides in a tubule, and the matrix forms around the cell processes.

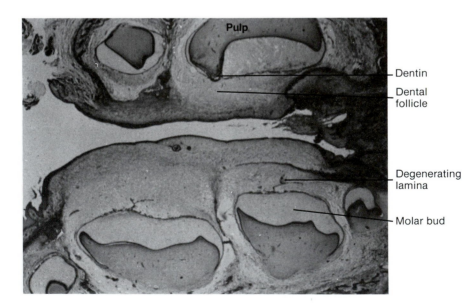

Figure 5.7 *Histology of tooth development, with a sagittal view of the maxillary and mandibular arches with molar tooth buds.*

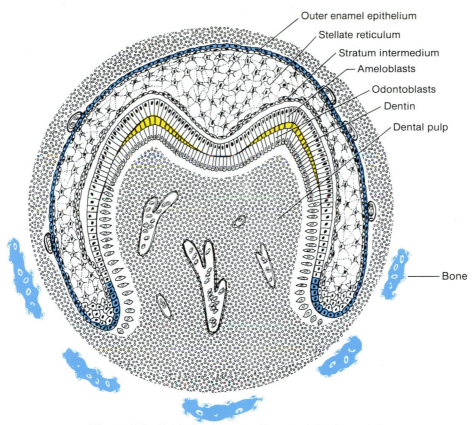

Outer enamel epithelium
Stellate reticulum
Stratum intermedium
Ameloblasts
Odontoblasts
Dentin
Dental pulp

Bone

Figure 5.8 *Tooth development. Diagram of dentinogenesis.*

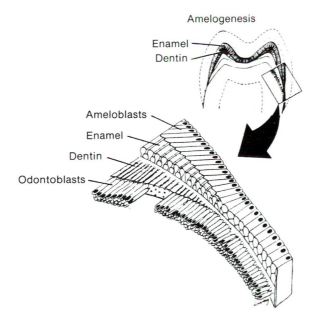

Amelogenesis

Enamel
Dentin

Ameloblasts
Enamel
Dentin
Odontoblasts

Figure 5.9 *Tooth development: ameloblasts and odontoblasts move away from the dentinoenamel junction (i.e, from each other), depositing enamel and dentin matrix.*

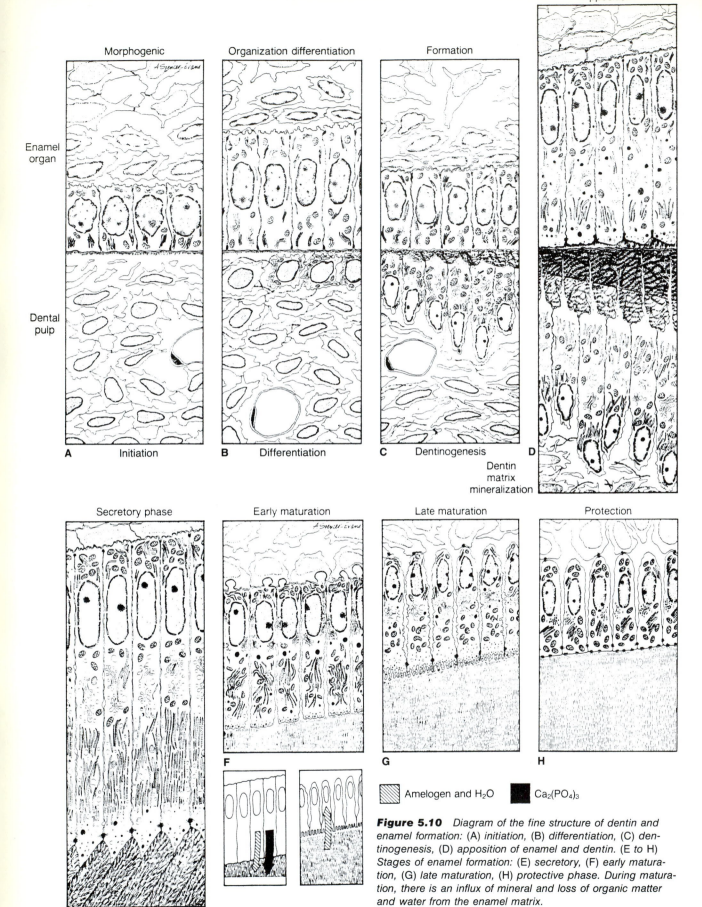

Morphogenic

Organization differentiation

Formation

Apposition

Enamel organ

Dental pulp

A Initiation

B Differentiation

C Dentinogenesis

Dentin matrix mineralization

D

Secretory phase

Early maturation

Late maturation

Protection

E

F

G

H

Amelogen and H₂O

Ca₂(PO₄)₃

Figure 5.10 *Diagram of the fine structure of dentin and enamel formation: (A) initiation, (B) differentiation, (C) dentinogenesis, (D) apposition of enamel and dentin. (E to H) Stages of enamel formation: (E) secretory, (F) early maturation, (G) late maturation, (H) protective phase. During maturation, there is an influx of mineral and loss of organic matter and water from the enamel matrix.*

Dentinogenesis takes place in two phases: the first is the formation of the collagenous matrix, and the second is the deposition of tricalcium phosphate (hydroxyapatite) crystals in this matrix. The initial calcification appears as crystals that are in vesicles on the surface and within the collagen fibrils (Figure 5.11). Crystals are oriented along the long axes of these fibrils, and they grow and spread, changing the predentin into dentin. Only the newly formed band of collagen matrix along the pulp is then uncalcified (Figure 5.12). The processes of matrix formation and mineralization, therefore, are closely related. Mineralization proceeds by a gradual increase in mineral density of the dentin. As each daily increment of predentin forms along the pulpal boundary, the adjacent more peripheral predentin, which is formed the previous day, mineralizes to become dentin (Figures 5.10 and 5.14).

During the period of crown development and tooth eruption, approximately 4 μm of dentin is formed daily. After the teeth reach occlusion and become functional, the rate of dentinal deposition decreases to less than 1 μm per day. The dentin formed each day is termed an **increment.** Increment means an addition of or increase in size, and the daily deposition is demarcated by microscopically visible lines in the hard tissue of teeth and bones. These lines are appropriately termed **incremental lines** (Figure 5.14). Incremental lines are believed to result from hesitation in matrix formation, resulting in lines of altered mineralization. The formative process is a daily rhythmic deposition. Incremental deposition and mineralization of dentin begin at the dentinoenamel junction and over the lateral areas of the crown and in the roots (Figure 5.15). Root development continues during and after tooth eruption (see Figure 5.1G).

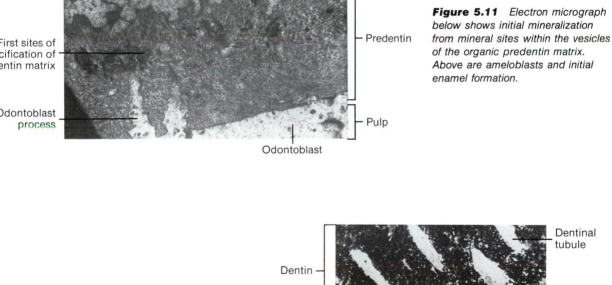

Ameloblast

First sites of calcification of dentin matrix

Odontoblast process

Forming enamel matrix

Predentin

Pulp

Odontoblast

Figure 5.11 *Electron micrograph below shows initial mineralization from mineral sites within the vesicles of the organic predentin matrix. Above are ameloblasts and initial enamel formation.*

Figure 5.12 *Dentinogenesis: calcified dentin seen above and predentin and odontoblasts below. Mineralization occurs along the dentin-predentin junction. Electron micrograph.*

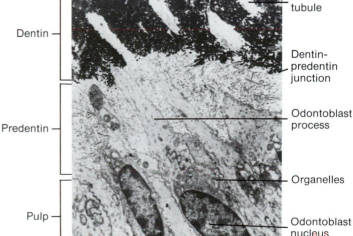

Dentin

Predentin

Pulp

Dentinal tubule

Dentin-predentin junction

Odontoblast process

Organelles

Odontoblast nucleus

■ *Amelogenesis*

Ameloblasts begin enamel deposition after a few micrometers of dentin have been deposited at the dentino-enamel junction (Figure 5.13). At the bell stage, cells of the inner enamel epithelium differentiate. They elongate and are ready to become active secretory ameloblasts. The ameloblasts then exhibit changes as they differentiate and pass through the functional stages of (1) morphogenesis, (2) organization and differentiation, (3) secretion, (4) maturation, and (5) protection (see Figure 5.10*A* to *H*).

The Golgi's apparatus appears centrally in the ameloblasts, and the amount of rough endoplasmic reticulum (RER) increases in the apical area (see Figure 5.10*D* and *E*). The row of ameloblasts maintains orientation by cell-to-cell attachments (desmosomes) at both the proximal and the distal ends of the cells. This maintains the cells in a row as they move peripherally from the dentinoenamel junction depositing enamel matrix (see Figure 5.9).

Short conical processes (**Tomes' processes**) develop at the apical end of the ameloblasts during the secretory stage (Figures 5.10*E* and 5.16). Junctional complexes appear at the junction of the cell bodies and Tomes' processes, called the **terminal bar apparatus,** and then they maintain contact between adjacent cells (Figure 5.10*E*). As the ameloblast differentiates, the matrix is synthesized within the rough endoplasmic reticulum, which then migrates to Golgi's apparatus, where it is condensed and packaged in membrane-bound granules. Vesicles migrate

to the apical end of the cell, where their contents are exteriorized and deposited first along the junction of the enamel and dentin (see Figure 5.16). This first enamel deposited on the surface of the dentin establishes the dentinoenamel junction. Figure 5.17 is an electron micrograph of young enamel matrix formed along the dentinoenamel junction. The Tomes' process of the ameloblast indents the surface of enamel (see Figures 5.10*E,* 5.16, and 5.17) until all the matrix has been deposited. Figure 5.18 illustrates how the surface of forming enamel rods can be seen. The forming enamel surface is pitted where the apical part of the cells (Tomes' process) is located in the enamel surface. The enamel matrix is formed in rods that are continuous from the dentinoenamel junction to the surface of the tooth.

When ameloblasts begin secretion, the overlying cells of the stratum intermedium enlarge and change from spindle to pyramidal shapes (see Figure 5.10*B* to *F*). The position of the cells during enamel production is closely related to their function in enamel formation, as are the ameloblasts. **Desmosome** attachment sites hold these two epithelial cell types in close proximity. Desmosomes are zones of attachment between two cells. Substances needed for enamel development arrive in the blood vessels in the outer enamel epithelium and next filter through the stellate reticulum to the stratum intermedium cells. These substances then pass to the ameloblasts, where synthesis of the enamel protein **amelogenin** occurs (see Figure 5.13).

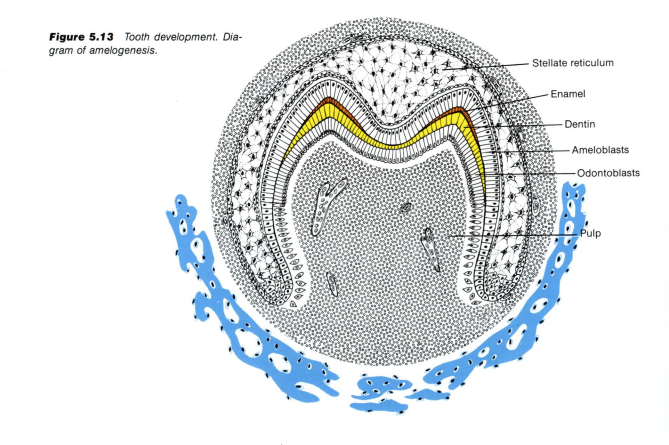

Figure 5.13   *Tooth development. Diagram of amelogenesis.*

Stellate reticulum

Enamel

Dentin

Ameloblasts

Odontoblasts

Pulp

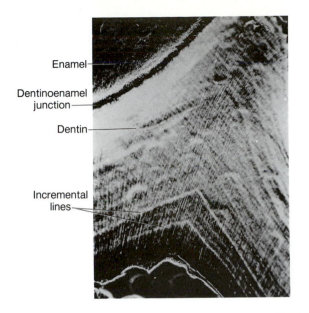

Figure 5.14 *Dentin microradiograph showing incremental lines in dentin.*

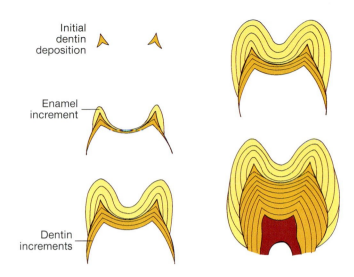

Figure 5.15 *The pattern of incremental dentin formation and enamel from initiation to completion. Begin at upper left crown to lower right.*

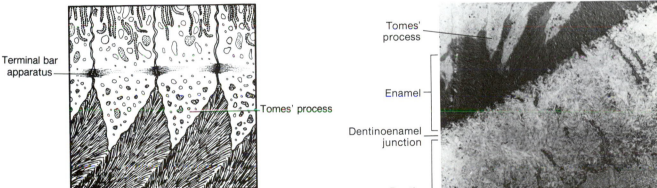

Figure 5.16 *Development of the Tomes' process of the ameloblast during amelogenesis.*

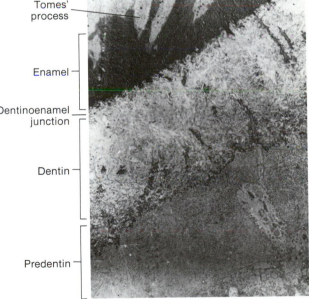

Figure 5.17 *Ultrastructure of the formation of the early enamel and dentin matrix at the dentinoenamel junction. Above is enamel, and below are dentin and predentin.*

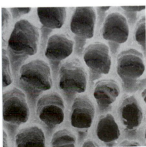

Human deciduous molar

Developing enamel surface

Height of field, 15–18 μm

Figure 5.18 *A scanning electron micrograph of the ameloblast–enamel matrix interface during amelogenesis.*

■ Crown Maturation

As soon as the amelogenin is deposited, the matrix beings to mineralize (see Figure 5.10F to H). The small crystals of mineral grow in length and diameter rapidly. Initial deposition of mineral amounts to approximately 25 percent of the total; 70 percent of the mineral in enamel is a result of further growth of the crystals (5 percent is water). The pattern of mineralization of enamel closely follows the pattern of matrix deposition. The first matrix deposited is the first enamel mineralized, occurring along the DEJ. Matrix formation and mineralization continue peripherally to the tips of the cusps and then laterally on the crowns (see Figure 5.15). Finally, the cervical region of each crown mineralizes. The protein of mature enamel is termed **enamelin.**

The mineral content of enamel rapidly surpasses that of dentin, which is about 69 percent. Enamel is composed of approximately 96 percent mineral, the largest concentration of mineral in any tissue of the body. Because of the high mineral content of enamel, almost all water and organic material are lost from it during maturation.

As the ameloblast completes the matrix deposition phase, its terminal bar apparatus disappears and the surface of the enamel becomes smooth (see Figure 5.10F and G). This phase is signaled by a change in the appearance as well as the function of the ameloblast. The apical end of this cell becomes ruffled along the enamel surface. The length of the ameloblast decreases, as does the number of organelles within it. The enamel has now reached the maturation phase, and the ameloblast becomes more active in absorption of the organic matrix and water from enamel, which allows mineralization to proceed (see Figure 5.10F to H).

■ Clinical Comment

The ameloblasts are remarkable cells because they first secrete and then calcify a matrix that becomes the hardest tissue in the body. For this to be accomplished, these cells must also resorb some of this matrix to allow final mineralization.

The increased mineral content in enamel is dependent on this loss of fluid and protein. This process of exchange occurs throughout much of enamel maturation and is not limited to this final stage. Even after the teeth erupt following birth, mineralization of enamel continues.

Finally, the ameloblasts secrete an organic cuticle on the surface of the enamel and then attach themselves to this organic covering of the tooth by **hemidesmosomes** (see Figure 5.10H). A hemidesmosome is half of a desmosome attachment plaque, and it relates to the attachment of a cell to a surface membrane rather than cell to cell as in a desmosome. Hemidesmosome attachment complex

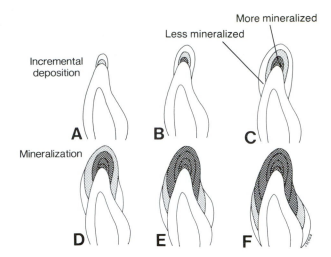

Figure 5.19 Summary of the stages of enamel mineralization. (A) Initial enamel is formed. (B) It is calcified, and further matrix is formed. (C) Further increments are formed. (D) Further matrix deposition and mineralization proceed. (E and F) Matrix is formed at sides and cervical area of the cusp.

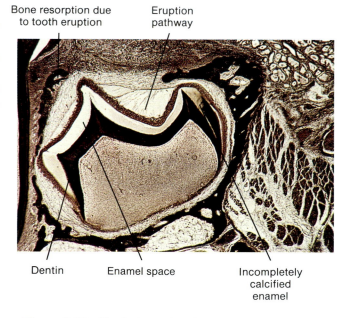

Figure 5.20 Histologic section of nearly mineralized enamel of the crown. The enamel matrix is seen only at the cervical region.

(plaques) is developed by the ameloblasts. This stage of cuticle formation is known as the protective phase of ameloblast function.

The thickness of enamel on the cusps is attained completely before the ameloblast completes enamel formation. The crowns are first, and the cervical region is the last area to form and to mineralize. Figure 5.19 illustrates the steps in enamel maturation. The cervical region is the last to mineralize and may be structurally deficient (Figure 5.20). This is believed to explain the susceptibility of this area to caries.

Growth of cusps to predetermined point of completion

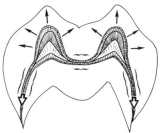

Figure 5.21 *Growth areas of a developing crown. Growth at cusp tip, intercuspal region, and cervical region.*

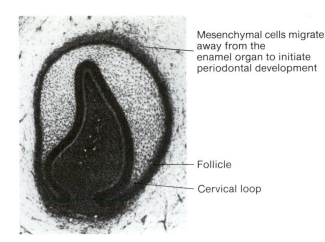

Mesenchymal cells migrate away from the enamel organ to initiate periodontal development

Follicle

Cervical loop

Figure 5.22 *Histology of an enamel organ at the bell stage of development with the cervical loop present. Mesenchymal cells on the surface of the enamel organ migrate peripherally and initiate development of the future periodontium.*

Crowns of teeth increase in size by additional incremental deposition of enamel matrix on the periphery of the cusps (see Figure 5.15). The first area of the crown to form completely is the cusp tip, and the last is the cervical region. Crowns also increase in size by cell proliferation of the inner enamel epithelial cells between cusps (Figure 5.21). Crowns increase in height or length by differentiation of new ameloblasts, followed by enamel formation in the cervical region of the forming crown. From the inception of enamel development to the completion of enamel formation, the crown increases in size about four times.

The completion of enamel is signaled by attainment of crown size and also by mineral content. Following the final stage of mineralization, the shortened ameloblasts secrete the **developmental** or **primary cuticle.**

■ Development of the Tooth Root

Root Sheath

As the crown develops, cell proliferation continues at the cervical region or base of the enamel organ, where the outer and inner enamel epithelial cells come together (Figure 5.22). This area is termed the **cervical loop.** When the crown is complete, these cells continue to lengthen, forming a double layer of cells termed the **epithelial root sheath,** or Hertwig's sheath (Figure 5.23A). In the crown, the inner cell layer becomes ameloblasts and functions in enamel formation, whereas in the root, these cells induce odontoblasts to form root dentin. The root sheath starts at the cementoenamel junction and continues to lengthen as the architect of the root. The length, curvature, thickness, and number of the roots are all dependent on these cells and their interaction with the adjacent pulp mesenchymal cells (Figure 5.23). While the inner root sheath cells stimulate the differentiation of odontoblasts and dentin formation, the outer root sheath cells then deposit a cuticular membrane (**enameloid**) on the surface of the root. Then the root sheath cells break down, and some migrate from the root

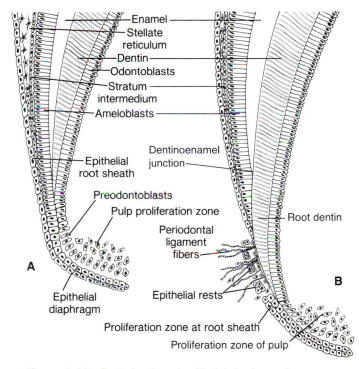

Enamel — Stellate reticulum — Dentin — Odontoblasts — Stratum intermedium — Ameloblasts —

Dentinoenamel junction —

Epithelial root sheath

Preodontoblasts

Pulp proliferation zone

Periodontal ligament fibers

Root dentin

A

B

Epithelial diaphragm

Epithelial rests

Proliferation zone at root sheath

Proliferation zone of pulp

Figure 5.23 *Root sheath and epithelial diaphragm formation. (A) Stage of initiation of the root sheath at the dentinoenamel junction. (B) In a later stage of root sheath development, root dentin is formed below the cervical enamel.*

surface (Figure 5.23B). At its advancing end, the root sheath bends pulpward at a near 45-degree angle. This area is termed the **epithelial diaphragm** (Figure 5.23A and B). The epithelial diaphragm therefore encircles the apical opening to the pulp during root development. It is the proliferation of these cells that accomplishes further growth of the root sheath and root.

As the root sheath lengthens, the odontoblasts differentiate along the pulpal boundary and root dentin proceeds. There is a continuation of dentin formation from the crown extending into the root (Figure 5.24). The dentin tapers from the crown to the apical epithelial diaphragm. In the root pulp, a large number of cells known as the **pulp proliferative zone** appear (see Figure 5.23A and B). This zone is believed to give rise to the new odontoblasts and fibroblasts of the pulp needed for the root to lengthen. Dentinogenesis continues until the root is completed, with an apical foramen measuring 1 to 3 mm. With increased root length, the tooth moves upward in the dental crypt to make space for further root growth. The root lengthens at the same rate as tooth eruptive movements occur (Figure 5.25).

■ Clinical Comment

The root sheath determines whether a tooth has single or multiple roots, is short or long, or is curved or straight. However, if there is insufficient space, roots conform to the space available.

Single Root

The root sheath of a single-rooted tooth is a tubelike growth of epithelial cells enclosing a tube of dentin and the developing pulp (see Figure 5.24). As soon as the root sheath cells deposit the enameloid, the root sheath breaks up, forming **epithelial rests** (Figures 5.23B and 5.26). The epithelial rests persist as they move away from the root surface into the follicular area. Mesenchymal cells from the follicular area then move between the epithelial cell rests to contact the root surface. Here, they differentiate into cementoblasts and begin secretion of **cementoid.** Cementoid is noncalcified cementum that soon mineralizes into mature cementum (Figure 5.27). The root sheath therefore is never seen as a continuous structure, since its cell layers break down rapidly once root dentin begins forming. However, the area of the epithelial diaphragm is maintained until the root is complete.

Multiple Roots

Multirooted teeth develop similarly to single-rooted teeth until the furcation zone begins to form (Figure 5.28). Division of the roots then takes place through differential growth of the root sheath. In two or more areas, the cells of the epithelial diaphragm grow excessively until they contact the opposing extensions (Figure 5.28). These extensions then fuse, and the original single opening is divided into two or three openings. The epithelial diaphragms surrounding the openings to each root then continue to grow at an equal rate. When a developing molar root is sectioned through, an area in the center of the root would show this root sheath

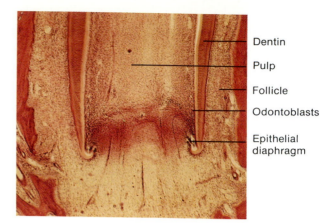

Figure 5.24   *Histology of root sheath and epithelial diaphragm. Observe the root dentin and highly cellular pulp.*

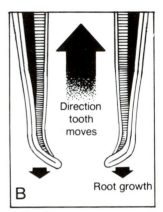

Figure 5.25   *The direction of root growth versus the eruptive movements of a tooth.*

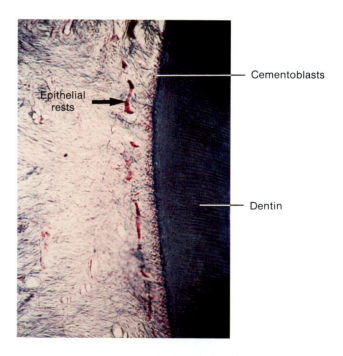

Figure 5.26   *Histologic micrograph of epithelial rests from the root sheath along the surface of root dentin.*

as an island of cells (Figure 5.29). As the multiple roots form, each root develops the same as a single-rooted tooth. After the root sheath breaks up and the epithelial rests move away from the root surface, cementum forms on the root surfaces. The cementum that forms near the cementoenamel junction appears acellular, whereas the cementum at the apex of the root, which is formed after tooth eruption, is cellular (Figure 5.30). Since the apical cementum is thicker, it probably requires the presence of cementocytes to maintain its vitality. The cementum is deposited like bone or dentin in successive layers or increments. Cementum may reach a quiescent stage, activating only in response to repair needs.

■ *Clinical Comment*

Growth of the jaws is necessary for the change from the primary to the permanent dentition. With the lengthening of the jaws, the permanent molars have space to develop and erupt. The jaws protect each tooth with a shell-like enclosure of bone.

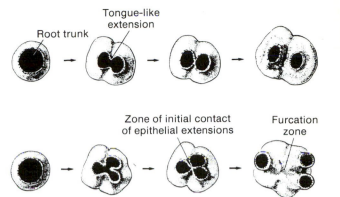

Figure 5.28 *Multiple-root development. Observe the extensions of the epithelial diaphragms as they make contact and fuse to divide a single root into two or three roots.*

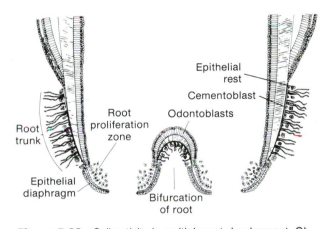

Figure 5.29 *Cell activity in multiple-root development. Observe the bifurcation zone. The root trunk is the common root area from the crown to the site of root bifurcation.*

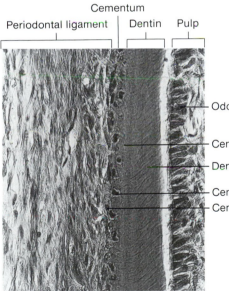

Figure 5.27 *Histologic micrograph of cellular cementum on the surface of dentin. Observe the cementocytes in the cementum and cementoblasts on the surface of the cementum. Periodontal ligament is on the left; pulp cells are on the right.*

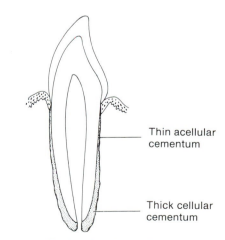

Figure 5.30 *The location of acellular cement in the cervical area and cellular cementum at the root apex.*

■ Development of Supporting Structures

The mesenchymal cells immediately surrounding the crown are known as the dental follicle (see Figure 5.22). Those folicular cells of mesenchymal origin lie adjacent to the young enamel organ during the cap and bell stages (see Figure 5.22). These cells then migrate from the enamel organ into the follicle, where they function in the formation of the alveolar bone and periodontal ligament. The future periodontal ligament is an area of connective tissue that surrounds the tooth, and it is positioned between the protective shell of alveolar bone and the developing tooth. Later, after tooth eruption, the periodontal ligament develops further and firmly attaches the teeth to the bone.

Periodontal Ligament

In addition to cementum, the periodontal ligament develops from the dental follicle and forms a specialized attachment between the cementum of the tooth and the alveolar bone. Delicate fibers first appear in the apical region of the roots when they initially begin formation in the cervical area. These are probably the stem cell fibroblasts that give rise to further fiber groups that appear as the roots elongate (Figure 5.31). As these fibers become embedded in the cementum at one end, the other end spreads out to contact the forming alveolar bone. There is evidence that these fibers turnover rapidly, and as the location of origin is established, they are continually renewed. Collagen turnover takes place throughout the ligament, although the highest turnover is in the apical area and the lowest in the cervical region. Maturation of the ligament, meaning increase in density, occurs as the teeth reach functional occlusion.

Alveolar Process

As the teeth develop, there is also development of the alveolar process to keep pace with the teeth's lengthening roots. At first, the alveolar process forms as a bony trench in which the tooth germs develop. This trench then deepens, and septa appear between each tooth to complete the crypts (Figure 5.32). When the teeth erupt, the alveolar process and periodontal ligament mature to support the functioning teeth (Figure 5.33). Bone that forms between the roots of multirooted teeth is termed **interradicular bone.** In the mature form, the alveolar bone is composed of the **alveolar bone proper** and the **supporting bone.** The former bone lines the tooth socket, and the latter is the supporting bone composed of both spongy and dense or compact supporting bone. This dense bone is the cortical plate covering the mandible (Figure 5.34).

■ Clinical Comment

Accessory root canals may connect the pulp with the periodontal ligament at any point along the root, although it usually appears near the apex. Pulp or periodontal infection can spread by means of this route to the adjacent tissue. A periodontal pocket resistant to treatment could be caused by this defect.

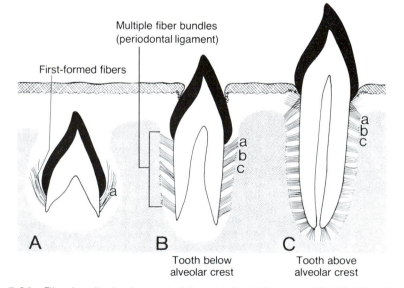

Multiple fiber bundles
(periodontal ligament)

First-formed fibers

A

B
Tooth below
alveolar crest

C
Tooth above
alveolar crest

Figure 5.31 *Fiber bundle development of the periodontal ligament. (A) Initial fiber formation; (B) secondary fibers develop; and (C) further fiber development, observe the change in direction of these initial fiber groups (A to C).*

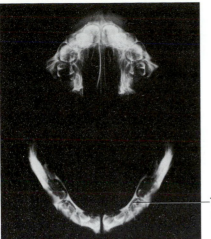

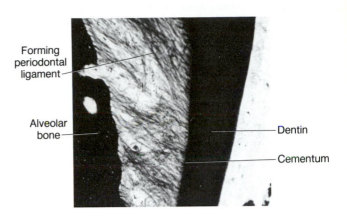

Figure 5.32 *Microradiograph of the maxillary and mandibular arches, illustrating the alveolar bone wih tooth crypts enclosing developing teeth in the prenatal embryo.*

Figure 5.33 *Appearance of the periodontal ligament fibers after tooth eruption. Observe the density of the fibers.*

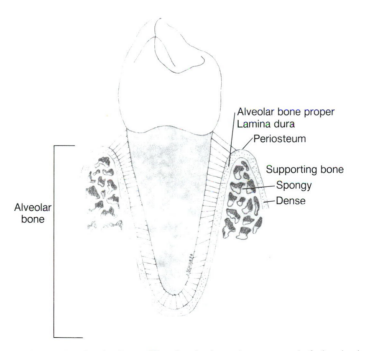

Figure 5.34 *A tooth in alveolar bone. The alveolar bone is composed of alveolar bone proper, which lines the socket and the supporting bone. The supporting bone is made up of spongy or cancellous bone and the dense or compact bone.*

In summary, in the simplest form, tooth development involves the interactive events of two types of oral tissues, epithelial and mesenchymal, which develop through the soft tissue stages of bud, cap, and bell. This is followed by the hard tissue formative stages of dentinogenesis and amelogenesis. Root formation logically follows crown de-

velopment. Each stage of development includes morphologic changes in shape and size, which are coordinated with microscopic changes in cell shape and function. Some of these relationships are seen in Figure 5.35.

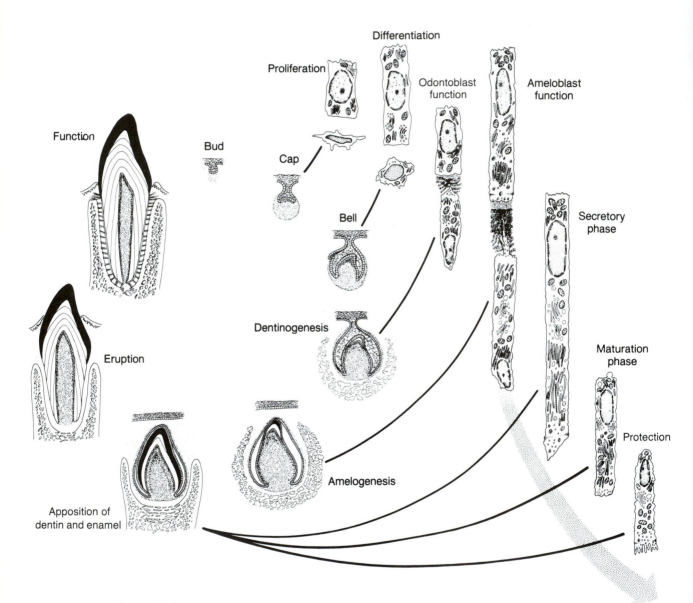

Figure 5.35 *Changes in the formative cells of the developing teeth are shown in the right diagrams and relate to the morphologic changes shown on the left. Cell proliferation relates to the cap stage, and cell differentiation relates to the bell stage. Odontoblast function relates to dentinogenesis and ameloblast function to amelogenesis. The labels* secretory phase, maturation phase, *and* protection *relate to the ameloblast function.*

■ Self-Evaluation Questions

1. What two cell types interact in tooth development?
2. Describe the two characteristics of the bell stage of tooth development.
3. List and define each stage of tooth development.
4. Describe the dental papilla. When does it become the pulp organ?
5. Describe the differentiation of the odontoblast and the initiation of dentin formation.
6. Why is dentinogenesis called a two-phase process?
7. What are the five stages of enamel formation?
8. What structure enables the ameloblasts to move in a row rather than individually during enamel formation?
9. What areas of the enamel are last to calcify in the crown?
10. Enamel completion is signaled by what two processes?

■ Acknowledgments

Dr. N.M. ElNesr contributed to the production of Chapter 8, Development of Root and Supporting Structures, in Avery, J.K., ed., *Oral Development and Histology,* Toronto: B.C. Decker, 1988. Some of the figures from that text have been used in this chapter.

■ Suggested Reading

Bhaskar, S.N., Development and growth of the teeth. In: Bhaskar, S.N. ed., Orban's oral histology and embryology. St. Louis: C.V. Mosby, 1986.

Lindskog, S. Morphology and formation of intermediate cementum in monkey (thesis). Stockholm: Karolinska Institute. 1982.

Ten Cate, A.R. Development of the periodontium. In: Ten Cate, A.R., ed. Oral histology, development, structure, and function. St. Louis: C.V. Mosby, 1989.

Ten Cate, A.R. Development of the tooth. In: Ten Cate, A.R., ed. Oral histology, development, structure, and function. St. Louis: C.V. Mosby, 1989.

6 · Eruption and Exfoliation of Teeth

■ Overview

Tooth eruption is the process by which developing teeth emerge through bone and soft tissue of the jaws and the overlying mucosa to enter the oral cavity, contact teeth of the opposing arch, and function in mastication. The movements related to tooth eruption begin during crown formation and require adjustments relative to the forming bony crypt. This is termed the **pre-eruptive phase.** Tooth eruption is also involved in the initiation of root development and continues until the tooth's emergence into the oral cavity, called the **prefunctional eruptive phase.** The teeth continue to erupt until they reach occlusal or incisal contact. Then they undergo functional eruptive movements, which include compensation for jaw growth and occlusal wear of the enamel. This stage is known as the **functional eruptive phase.** Eruption is actually a continuous process, ending only with the loss of the tooth. Each dentition, primary and permanent, has various problems during eruption and in the sequencing of eruption in the oral cavity. Teeth differ extensively in their eruptive schedules as well.

These various events are described in this chapter. Finally, the process of tooth exfoliation is presented. The three causes that function in primary tooth loss by exfoliation are noted.

■ *Pre-eruptive Phase*

The pre-eruptive phase of tooth eruption includes all movements of the primary and permanent tooth crowns from the time of their early initiation and formation to the time of crown completion. Therefore, this phase is finished with the initiation of root development. Throughout the pre-eruptive phase, the developing crowns move constantly in the jaws. They respond to positional changes of the neighboring crowns and the changes in the mandible and maxilla as the face develops outward, forward, and downward away from the brain in its maturing growth path. During the lengthening of the jaws, there are mesial and distal movements of both the primary and permanent teeth. Eventually, the permanent tooth crowns move within the jaws, adjusting their position to the resorptive roots of the primary dentition and the remodeling alveolar process, especially during the mixed dentition period from 8 to 12 years of age.

Early in the pre-eruptive period, the permanent anterior teeth begin developing lingual to and near the incisal level of their primary predecessors (Figures 6.1 and 6.2). Later, however, as the primary teeth erupt, the permanent successors are positioned lingual to and near the apical third of their roots. The permanent premolars shift from a location near the occlusal area of the primary molars to a location beneath and enclosed within the roots of the primary molars (Figure 6.2). This change in relative position is due to the eruption of the primary teeth and an increase in height of the supporting structures. On the other hand, the permanent molars, which have no primary predecessors, develop without this type of relationship (Figure 6.3). The maxillary molars develop within the tuberosities of the maxilla, with their occlusal surfaces slanting distally. The mandibular molars develop in the mandibular rami, with their occlusal surfaces slanting mesially (see Figure 6.3). This slant is due to their angle of eruption as they arise from the curvature of the condyle of the posterior mandible. All movements in the pre-eruptive phase occur within the crypts of the developing and growing crown before root formation begins.

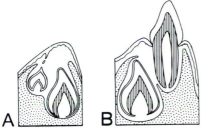 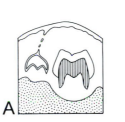 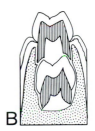

Figure 6.1 *The relative position of primary and permanent incisor teeth in (A) pre-eruptive and (B) prefunctional eruptive periods.*

Figure 6.2 *The relative position of primary molar and permanent premolar teeth in (A) pre-eruptive and (B) prefunctional eruptive periods.*

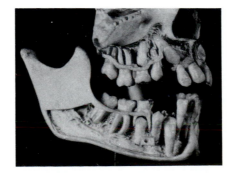

Figure 6.3 *Human jaws at 8 to 9 years of age, during the mixed dentition period. The permanent teeth are replacing the primary teeth. Observe the positions of each. The permanent mandibular molar has not emerged from the coronoid process.*

■ Prefunctional Eruptive Phase

The prefunctional eruptive phase starts with the initiation of root formation and ends when the teeth reach occlusal contact. Four major events occur during this phase.

1. **Root formation** occurs, requiring space for the elongation of the roots. The first step in root formation is a proliferation of the epithelial root sheath, which in time causes the initiation of root dentin and formation of the pulp tissue of the forming root. Root formation also causes an increase in the fibrous tissue of the surrounding dental follicle (Figure 6.4).

2. **Movement** is the second step of the erupting tooth. This action occurs incisally or occlusally through the bony crypt of the jaws to reach the oral mucosa. This movement is due to a need for the elongating roots to have space to form. The reduced enamel epithelium covering the enamel next contacts and fuses with the oral epithelium (Figure 6.5). Both of these epithelial cell layers proliferate toward each other, and their cells intermingle, and a fusion occurs between the reduced enamel and the oral epithelium. The reduced enamel epithelium gives rise to a thin epithelial layer overlying the erupting crown (Figure 6.6).

3. **Penetration** of the crown's tip through the fused epithelial layer is the next step. This action allows entrance of the enamel into the oral cavity. Only the organic developmental cuticle (primary), secreted earlier by the ameloblasts, then covers the enamel (Figure 6.7).

4. **Intraoral occlusal** or **incisal movement** of the erupting tooth continues until clinical contact with the opposing crown occurs. The crown moves farther through the mucosa causing a gradual exposure of more crown surface, with an increasingly apical shift of the gingival attachment (Figure 6.7). This exposed crown is termed the **clinical crown,** and it extends from the cusp tip to the area of the gingival attachment. In contrast, the **anatomic crown** is the entire crown extending from the cusp tip to the cementoenamel junction.

■ Clinical Comment

Hypereruption occurs when there is loss of an apposing tooth. This condition allows the tooth or teeth to erupt farther than normal into the space.

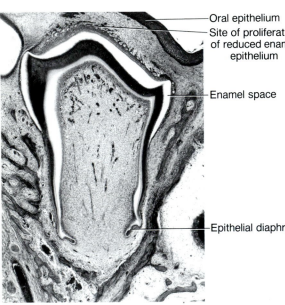

Oral epithelium

Site of proliferation of reduced enamel epithelium

Enamel space

Epithelial diaphragm

Figure 6.4 *Histology of the prefunctional eruptive phase. The root is developing, and reduced epithelium overlying the crown approaches the oral mucosa. Note proliferation of the epithelium.*

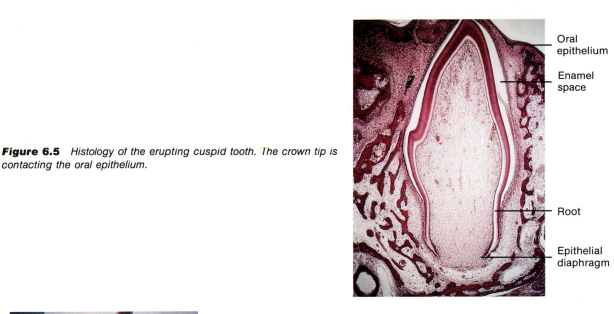

Figure 6.5 *Histology of the erupting cuspid tooth. The crown tip is contacting the oral epithelium.*

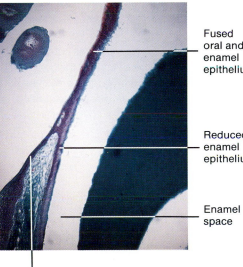

Figure 6.6 *Histology of the erupting tooth. Fused enamel and oral epithelium are stretched over the enamel. (Enamel is dissolved in preparation, creating the enamel space.)*

Figure 6.7 *Histology of the erupting primary tooth and appearance of the clinical crown in the mouth. Observe the position of the permanent tooth on the left. Dotted line indicates cuticle overlying enamel surface of erupting tooth.*

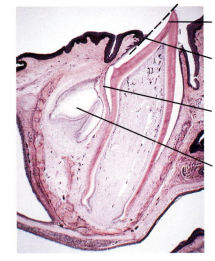

Changes in Tissues

The prefunctional eruptive phase is characterized by significant changes that take place in the tissues **overlying, surrounding,** and **underlying** the erupting teeth.

Overlying the Teeth

The dental follicle becomes altered, forming a pathway for the erupting teeth. There first appears a zone of degenerating connective tissue fibers and cells immediately overlying the teeth (Figures 6.8 and 6.9). During this process, blood vessels decrease in number and nerve fibers break into pieces and degenerate. The altered tissue space or compartment overlying the teeth becomes visible as an inverted triangular area, known as the **eruption pathway.** In the periphery of this zone, the follicular fibers, regarded as the **gubernaculum dentis** or **gubernacular cord** (Figure 6.10), are directed toward the mucosa. Some authors believe that these fibers guide the teeth in eruptive movements to ensure complete tooth eruption.

Macrophages appear in the soft tissue. These cells cause the release of hydrolytic enzymes that aid in the destruction of tissues in this area and the loss of blood vessels. Osteoclasts are found along the borders of the resorptive bone overlying the teeth. This loss of bone overlying the teeth keeps pace during eruptive movement (see Figure 6.9). **Osteoclasts** and **osteoblasts** constantly remodel the bone as the tooth enlarges and moves along in the direction of the growing face (see Figure 6.9). Tooth eruption along with the increased amount of supporting alveolar bone can be considered part of the height increase for the developing face.

Although eruption of permanent teeth is similar to that of primary teeth, the presence of the primary tooth roots presents an additional problem. The need for resorption of their roots is similar to the process of bone resorption for the emergence of primary teeth. Permanent teeth establish an eruptive path lingual to the primary anterior teeth and the premolars under the primary molars. The permanent molars erupt into the free alveolar space behind the primary teeth (see Figure 6.9). Small foramina in the mandible and maxilla just posterior to the primary tooth row are evidence of the eruption sites of the anterior permanent teeth (Figure 6.11). As the roots resorb, the primary crowns are lost, which is known as **exfoliation** of teeth (Figure 6.12). Dentin resorption is similar to bone resorption.

The resorptive process of teeth or bone results from the action of osteoclasts that arise from monocytes of the circulating blood stream. These monocytes appear and fuse with others to form the multicelled osteoclasts. Their function is to resorb the hard tissue. They do so by first separating the mineral from the collagen matrix. This is effected by the action of the hydrolytic enzymes secreted by the osteoclasts. This enzymatic action is believed to occur within lacunae, which are developed by the osteoclast. The osteoclast's cell membrane then contacts the bone (Figure 6.13). The cell membrane is modified by an enfolding area termed the **ruffled border.** This increases the surface area of the cell and allows the cell to maximally function in bone resorption (Figure 6.14).

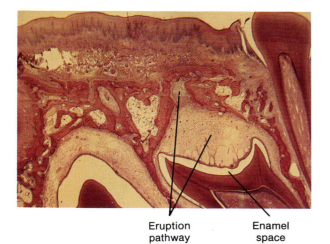

Eruption   Enamel
pathway   space

Figure 6.8   *Histology of the prefunctional erupting tooth. Observe the appearance of the eruption pathway overlying the crown.*

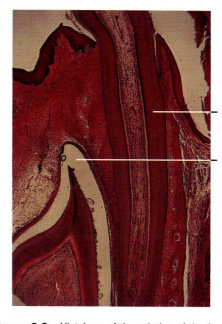

— Primary
  tooth

— Erupting
  permanent
  tooth
  crown

Figure 6.9   *Histology of the relation of the functional primary tooth root on the right to the permanent crown nearing eruption seen on the left.*

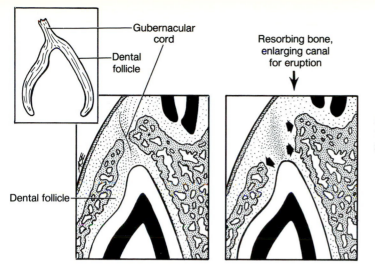

Figure 6.10 The developing eruption pathway. (A) The gubernaculum dentis. (B) Bone resorption from the eruption pathway.

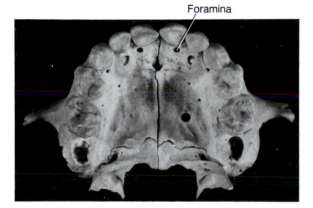

Figure 6.11 Maxillary foramina lingual to the primary incisors. These are the sites for eruption of the permanent incisors.

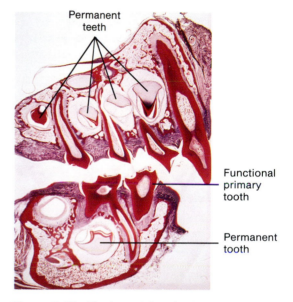

Figure 6.12 Histology of the mixed dentition period. Observe the erupted primary teeth above with the resorbing roots. Below are the crowns of the developing permanent teeth.

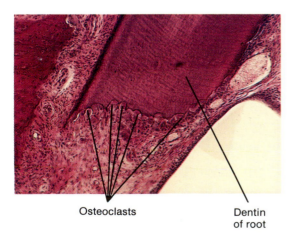

Figure 6.13 Histology of active resorption sites of primary tooth roots. Observe the osteoclasts in lacunae.

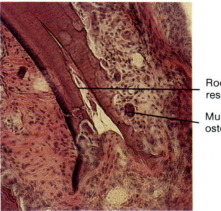

Figure 6.14 Histology of osteoclasts in resorption lacunae. Observe the large multinucleated cells within the lacunae.

Hard tissue resorption is believed to occur in two phases: the **extracellular phase,** in which the mineral is separated from the collagen and broken into small fragments (Figure 6.15), and the **intracellular phase,** in which the osteoclast ingests these mineral fragments and continues the dissolution of this mineral. Crystals appear in cytoplasmic vacuoles of the osteoclast and are gradually digested within them. Resorption of the mineral occurs at the ruffled border interface outside the cell and the mineral is then taken within the cell (Figure 6.16). Special fibroblast (**fibroblast-fibroclast**) cells are believed to secondarily destroy the remaining collagen fibers by ingesting them in an intracellular phagolysosome system (Figure 6.17). From this breakdown, resulting amino acids will be used in the formation of collagen, within this same cell, and will possibly be used in this same area for bone formation. Only the posterior permanent molars have no primary predeciduous teeth and therefore erupt only through alveolar bone (Figure 6.18).

Figure 6.19 summarizes what happens in the tissues overlying the teeth during their prefunctional eruptive phase. Bone loss is seen in Figure 6.19A. Contact of the overlying oral mucosa by the tooth is seen in Figure 6.19B and C. This contact causes a stretching and thinning of the oral membrane and finally its rupture and penetration by the tooth as depicted in Figure 6.19D and E. The tooth is only then covered with the thin developmental cuticle, which can be observed in Figure 6.19E and F. As the tooth emerges farther into the mouth, more crown is exposed, and as a clinical contact with the opposing tooth is made, the epithelial attachment shifts to the cervical area, as noted in Figure 6.19G. Clinically, tooth eruption is seen as a blanching of the mucosa, and this condition may persist for several days since the eruptive process is neither rapid nor continuous. Each eruptive movement, however, results in greater exposure of the crown, and with successive eruptive movements the area of attached epithelium becomes lower on the clinical crown.

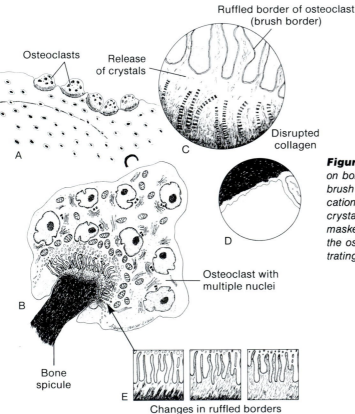

Figure 6.15 *Osteoclast activity. (A) Osteoclasts in lacunae on bone surface. (B) A large multinucleated osteoclast with brush border in contact with a bone spicule. (C) High magnification of the ruffled border of the osteoclast showing mineral crystals passing into spaces between cell extensions. Unmasked collagen fibers are nearby. (D) Clear zone seen on the osteoclast surface. (E) Ruffled border of osteoclast illustrating that it is in constant motion (change).*

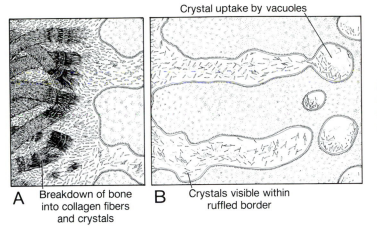

Crystal uptake by vacuoles

A — Breakdown of bone into collagen fibers and crystals

B — Crystals visible within ruffled border

Figure 6.16 (A) *High magnification of unmasked collagen fibers. Mineral crystals are near the osteoclast surface.* (B) *Diagram of the uptake of crystals into osteoclast vacuoles.*

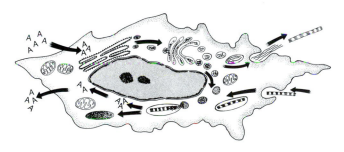

Figure 6.17 *A fibroblast (fibroblast-fibroclast) capable of synthesis of collagen as well as breakdown. Collagen fibers are phagocytized into cells and broken down to release amino acids. These amino acids are then used to form new collagen units.*

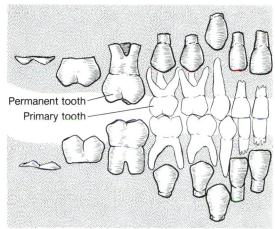

Permanent tooth
Primary tooth

Figure 6.18 *The relationship between primary and permanent teeth during the mixed dentition period.*

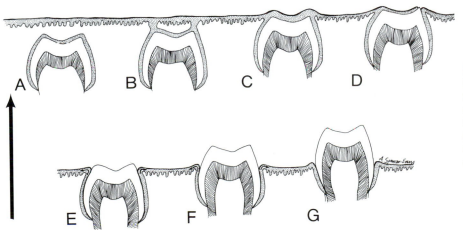

Figure 6.19 *Tooth eruption.* (A) *Crown penetrating bone and connective tissue.* (B) *Contact of crown with oral epithelium.* (C) *Fusion of epithelia.* (D) *Thinning of epithelia.* (E) *Rupture of epithelium.* (F) *Crown emergence.* (G) *Occlusal contact.*

Surrounding the Teeth

The tissues around the teeth change from delicate fibers lying parallel to the surface of the tooth to bundles of fibers attached to the tooth surface and extending toward the periodontium. The first fibers to appear are those in the cervical area as root formation begins (Figure 6.20A). As the root elongates further, bundles of fibers appear on the root surface (Figure 6.20B and C). Fibroblasts are the active cells in the formation and degradation of the collagen fibers. With tooth eruption, the alveolar bone of the crypt increases in height to accommodate the forming root. After the teeth attain functional occlusion, the fibers gain their mature orientation (Figure 6.21). Special fibroblasts have been reported in the periodontium of the erupting teeth. These **myofibroblasts** have contractile properties. During eruption, collagen formation and fiber turnover are very rapid, occurring within 24 hours. This mechanism enables fibers to attach and release and reattach in rapid succession. Some fibers may detach and later reattach while the tooth moves occlusally as new bone forms around the tooth. Gradually, the fibers organize, increasing in numbers and density as the tooth erupts in the oral cavity. Blood vessels then become more prominent in the developing ligament and exert additional pressure on the erupting tooth (Figure 6.21).

◼ *Clinical Comment*

Teeth are considered *submerged* when eruption is prevented because of crowding or tipping of the adjacent teeth into the space created by a missing tooth. *Retained primary teeth* may be due to lack of development of the permanent successor.

Underlying the Teeth

As the crown of a tooth begins to erupt, it gradually moves occlusally, providing space underlying the tooth for the root to lengthen (Figure 6.22). In the fundic region, these changes in the soft tissue and bone surrounding the root apex are believed to be largely compensatory to the lengthening of the root. During root formation, the dentin of the root apex tapers to a fine point that terminates in the epithelial diaphragm (Figure 6.23). Fibroblasts form collagen along the root apex, and these fiber bundles become attached in the cementum as it forms on the dentin near the apex. Fibroblasts appear in great numbers in the fundic area, and some of these fibers in the nearby area form fine strands of fibers that soon are calcified into bony trabeculae. These trabeculae form a network, or bony ladderlike arrangement, at the tooth apex, which is believed to fill the space and compensate for the eruptive movements of the teeth (Figure 6.23). Gradually, the delicate bone ladder becomes denser as additional bony plates appear (see Figure 6.22). These bony plates are maintained until the teeth reach occlusion at the end of this phase. Dense bone then forms around the tooth's apex, and bundles of fibers attach to the apical cementum and the alveolar bone to further support the tooth (Figure 6.24).

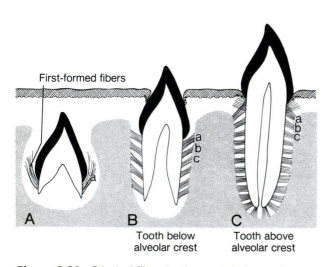

Figure 6.20 *Principal fiber development during tooth eruption. (A) Origin of fibers at the cervical area. (B) Further fiber development with root growth. (C) Change in orientation of the fibers with occlusal function. (a) Initial fiber formation. (b) Secondary fibers develop. (c) Further fiber development. Observe the changes in direction of these initial fiber groups.*

First-formed fibers

A   B   C

Tooth below alveolar crest

Tooth above alveolar crest

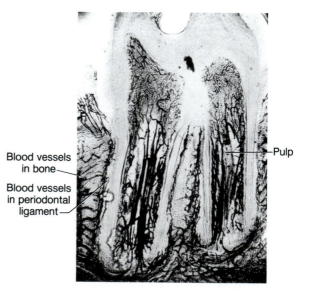

Blood vessels in bone

Blood vessels in periodontal ligament

Pulp

Figure 6.21 *Histology of the erupting tooth with vascular injection to illustrate presence of blood vessels in the periodontium and pulp.*

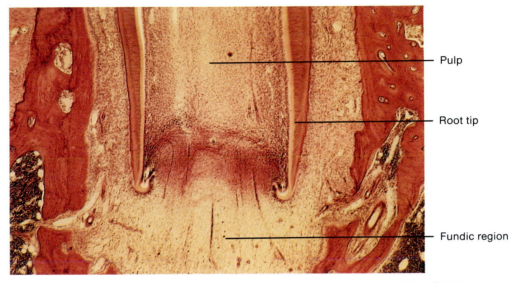

— Pulp

— Root tip

— Fundic region

Figure 6.22 *Histology of erupting tooth with immature roots and wide-open apices. As the tooth erupts, a bone ladder fills in the fundic region of the socket.*

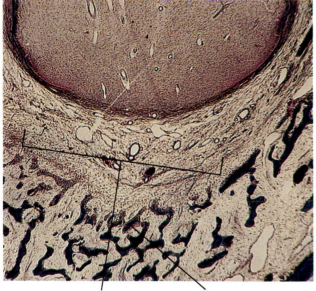

Zone of
cell proliferation

Bone of
fundic
region

Figure 6.23 *Histology of changes in the fundic region during tooth eruption. Fine trabeculae of new bone appear near tooth apices.*

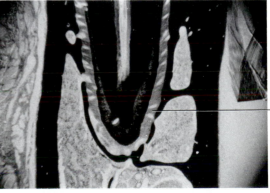

Periodontal
fiber
bundles

Figure 6.24 *Histology of the tooth in functional occlusion to show the density of functioning bundles of periodontal fibers. Note spaces between fiber bundles for blood vessels and nerves.*

■ Functional Eruptive Phase

The final eruptive phase takes place after the teeth are in function and continues as long as the teeth are present in the mouth. During this period of root completion, there is a compensating increase in the height of the alveolar process. The fundic alveolar plates resorb to adjust for formation of the root tip apex. The root canal narrows as a result of root tip maturation, at which time apical fibers develop to help cushion the forces of occlusal impact. Root completion continues for a considerable length of time, even after the teeth begin to function. This process takes about 1 to 1.5 years for deciduous teeth and 2 to 3 years for permanent teeth.

The most marked changes occur as occlusion is established. At that time, the mineral density of the alveolar bone increases and the principal fibers of the periodontal ligament increase in dimension and change orientation in their mature state. These fibers separate into groups oriented about the gingiva, the alveolar crest, and the alveolar surface around the root. Such fibers stabilize the tooth to a greater degree, and the blood vessels become more highly organized in spaces between bundles of fibers (Figure 6.24). Later in life, attrition and abrasion may wear down the occlusal or incisal surface of the teeth, causing the teeth to erupt slightly to compensate for this loss of tooth structure. Any such change results in deposition of cementum on the root's apex (Figure 6.25). Cementum is also deposited in the furcation area of a two- or three-rooted tooth.

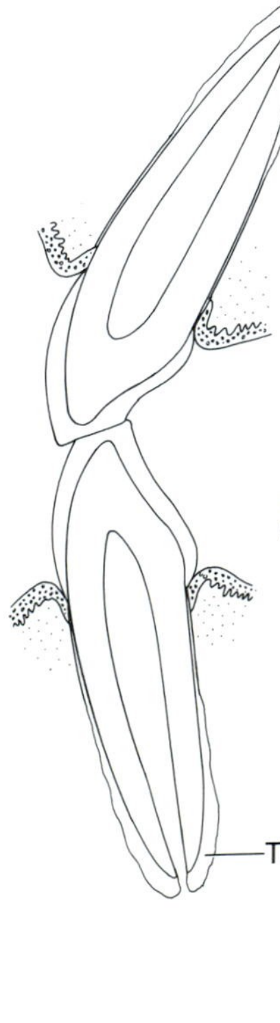

■ Possible Causes of Tooth Eruption

Of the numerous causes of tooth eruption, the most frequently cited are root growth and pulpal pressure. Other important causes are cell proliferation, increased vascularity, and increased bone formation around the teeth. Additional possible causative agents which have been noted include: endocrine influence, vascular changes, and enzymatic degradation. Probably all of these factors have an influencing role but not necessarily independently of each other.

Although all the factors associated with tooth eruption are not yet known, elongation of the root and modification of the alveolar bone and periodontal ligament are thought the most important factors. These events are coupled with the changes overlying the tooth that produce the eruption pathway. Blood vessels in this area are compressed by the advancing crown and become nonfunctional. Connective tissue in the eruption pathway gradually disappears, and the tooth epithelium and oral epithelium fuse. In summary, the erupting tooth moves from an area of increased pressure into an area of decreased pressure.

■ Clinical Comment

A lack of eruption may be related to fusion of tooth roots to the bony socket or to the crown of a permanent tooth. This condition is known as *ankylosis*, since there is fusion of the tooth root with underlying hard tissue.

■ Sequence and Chronology of Tooth Eruption

The formula for the eruptive sequence of the primary and permanent dentition appears in Table 6.1. The chronological development and eruption of the primary dentition is shown in Table 6.2, and that of the permanent dentition appears in Table 6.3.

Posteruptive changes: attrition and formation of compensatory cementum

Thickened cementum

Figure 6.25 *Functional eruptive changes illustrating attrition of the surface of enamel and compensatory deposition of cementum in the apical region.*

Table 6.1   The Sequence of Tooth Eruption

Primary

CI	LI	1M	Cu	2M
L	U	U	U	L
U	L	L	L	U

Permanent

U1M	LCI	UL	LCU	U1Pre	U2Pre	UCu	L2M	L3M
L1M	UCI	LL		L1Pre	L2Pre		U2M	U3M

Table 6.2   Chronology of Development of the Primary Dentition*

Primary teeth listed in order of eruption (sequence)	Beginning calcification (mo in utero)	Crown completed postnatally (mo)	Appearance in the oral cavity (eruption time) (mo)	Root completed time (yr)
Lower central incisor	3–4	2–3	6–8	1–2
Upper central incisor	3–4	2	7–10	1–2
Upper lateral incisor	4	2–3	8–11	2
Lower lateral incisor	4	3	9–13	1–2
Upper first molar	4	6	12–15	2–3
Lower first molar	4	6	12–16	2–3
Upper canine	4–5	9	16–19	3
Lower canine	4–5	9	17–20	3
Lower second molar	5	10	20–26	3
Upper second molar	5	11	25–28	3

* The normal range of eruption times indicates a wide variation in eruption times. It is important to know that a difference of 1 or 2 months either side of the normal range does not necessarily indicate that a child's eruption time schedule is abnormal. Only deviations considerably out of this range should be considered abnormal.

Table 6.3   Chronology of Development of the Permanent Dentition

Permanent teeth listed in order of eruption (sequence)	Beginning calcification	Crown completed (yr)	Appearance in the oral cavity (eruption time) (yr)	Root completed time (yr)
Lower first molar	Birth	3–4	6–7	9–10
Upper first molar	Birth	4–5	6–7	9–10
Lower central incisor	3–4 mo	4	6–7	9
Upper central incisor	3–4 mo	4–5	7–8	10
Lower lateral incisor	3–4 mo	4–5	7–8	9–10
Upper lateral incisor	10–12 mo	4–5	8–9	10–11
Lower canine	4–5 mo	5–6	9–10	12–13
Upper first premolar	1–2 yr	6–7	10–11	12–14
Lower first premolar	1–2 yr	6–7	10–11	12–14
Upper second premolar	2–3 yr	7–8	10–12	13–14
Lower second premolar	2–3 yr	7	11–12	14–15
Upper canine	4–5 mo	6–7	11–12	14–15
Lower second molar	2–3 yr	7–8	11–12	14–15
Upper second molar	2–3 yr	7–8	12–13	15–16
Lower third molar	8–10 yr	12–16	17–20	18–25
Upper third molar	7–9 yr	12–16	18–20	18–25

■ *Shedding of Primary Teeth*

Humans are considered **diphyodont** because they possess two dentitions, a primary and a permanent set. Teeth in the primary dentition are smaller and fewer than in the permanent dentition to conform with the small jaws of the infant. Teeth in the permanent dentition are larger and more numerous to accommodate the larger jaws of the adult.

The primary dentition functions for a brief period, from about two to eight years of age. When teeth from both dentitions are present, the period is one of **mixed dentition,** which extends from about eight to twelve years of age. This is an interesting period because only part of the primary tooth roots are present since they are undergoing resorption and only parts of the permanent roots are present since they are just forming. In this way, nearly 50 teeth can be present in the jaws during this four-year period (see Figure 6.12).

The period of tooth shedding follows mixed dentition. **Shedding** is the loss of the primary dentition owing to the physiologic resorption of the roots, loss of the supporting structures, and the increased masticatory forces required.

The degeneration of primary pulp tissue is similar to that of the tissues in the eruption pathway, with a loss of cells, fibers, nerves, and finally blood vessels (see Figure 6.12). When a primary tooth is extracted, blood is likely to still be in that crown, although only epithelium holds the tooth in the socket. Figure 6.26 shows the correlation between root growth and eruption. It illustrates changes that occur in the pre-eruptive, prefunctional, and functional eruptive stages, overlying and around the root surface as the tooth moves into function.

■ *Clinical Comment*

Teeth are considered *submerged* when eruption is prevented because of crowding or tipping of the adjacent teeth into the space created by a missing tooth. *Retained primary teeth* may be due to lack of development of the permanent successor.

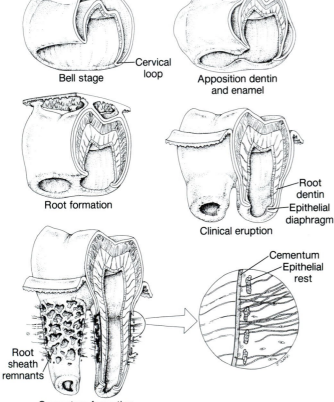

Bell stage — Cervical loop

Apposition dentin and enamel

Root formation

Clinical eruption — Root dentin — Epithelial diaphragm

Cementum — Epithelial rest

Root sheath remnants

Cementum formation

Figure 6.26 *Summary of tooth eruption. (A) Early pre-eruptive changes in the enamel organ at the bell stage. (B) Late pre-eruptive changes as the enamel and dentin form. (C) Early prefunctional changes as the tooth moves to the oral epithelium. (D) Late prefunctional change as the tooth emerges into the oral cavity. (E) Functional eruptive phase with clinical contact. Root growth is shown with the root sheath detaching from the root surface. Epithelial rests and cementum formation by cementoblasts are seen.*

■ Self-Evaluation Questions

1. What is the origin of osteoclasts?
2. Define tooth eruption and its three phases.
3. Describe the changes occurring around the tooth during eruption.
4. Describe the changes occurring in the area overlying the tooth during eruption.
5. Explain any significant changes occurring in the area underlying the tooth during eruption.
6. What are three causes of the shedding of primary teeth?
7. What phases occur in hard tissue resorption?
8. Give the sequence of eruption for the primary and permanent teeth.
9. Give the chronology of eruption for the primary and permanent teeth.
10. What enzymes contribute to the process of resorption for bone, dentin, and cementum?

■ Acknowledgment

Dr. N.M. Einesr contributed to the production of Chapter 10, Tooth Eruption and Shedding, in Avery, J.K., ed. *Oral Development and Histology,* Toronto: B.C. Decker, 1988. With appreciation, some of the comments and figures from that text have been used in this chapter.

■ Suggested Reading

Cahill, D.R. Histologic changes in the bony crypt and gubernacular canal erupting permanent premolars during deciduous premolar exfoliation in beagles. J. Dent. Res. 1974; 53:786.

Cahill, D.R., and Marks, S.C., Jr. Tooth eruption: Evidence for the central role of the dental follicle. J. Oral Pathol. 1980; 9:189.

Schroeder, H.E, and Listgarten, M.A. Fine structure of the developing epithelial attachment of human teeth. *In:* Wolsky, A., ed. Monographs in developmental biology, vol. 2. Basel: S. Karger, 1971.

Ten Cate, A.R., and Mills, C. The development of the periodontium: The origin of alveolar bone. Anat. Rec. 1972; 173:69.

Enamel

■ Overview

Enamel, a hard protective substance that covers the tooth surface, is the hardest biologic tissue in the human body. Consequently, it is able to resist fractures during the stress of mastication. Enamel provides the shape and contour for the crowns of teeth and covers that part of the tooth exposed to the oral environment.

Enamel is composed of interlocking rods that resist masticatory forces. Enamel rods are deposited in a keyhole shape by the formative ameloblastic cells. Groups of ameloblasts migrate from the dentinoenamel junction peripherally as they form these rods. Ameloblasts take variable paths, which produces a bending of the rods. These cells maintain a relationship as they travel in different directions producing adjacent rods. The enamel rod configuration, when viewed in incidental light, appears as light and dark bands of rod groups termed **Hunter-Schreger bands.** Because these rods bend in an exaggerated twisted manner at the cusp tips, they are called **gnarled enamel.**

All enamel rods are deposited in a daily appositional rate or increment of 4 μ. Such increments are noticeable, like rings of a tree in a longitudinal section, and appear as dark lines known as **striae of Retzius.** The growth lines become apparent on the surface of the enamel as ridges, known as perikymata. Two structures are noticeable at the dentinoenamel junction: spindles, the terminations of dentinal tubules in enamel, and tufts, hypocalcified zones caused by the bending of the adjacent groups of rods.

Since enamel is composed of bending rods, which in turn are composed of crystals, there are minute spaces or gaps where crystals did not form between rods. This feature causes enamel to be variable in its density and hardness. Therefore, some areas of enamel may differ in the ability to allow small particles to penetrate the enamel. This characteristic leads to tooth destruction by dental caries. After enamel is completely formed, there can be no further deposition of enamel.

■ Physical Properties

Because enamel is very hard, it is also brittle and subject to fracture. Fracture occurs especially if the underlying dentin is carious, causing a weak foundation.

Enamel is composed of more than 96 percent inorganic mineral in the form of **hydroxyapatite** and 4 percent water and organic matter. The hydroxyapatite is a crystalline calcium phosphate that is also found in bone, dentin, and cementum. The organic component of enamel is the protein **enamelin,** which is similar to the protein keratin found in the skin. The distribution of enamelin between and on the crystals of enamel aids enamel's semipermeability.

Enamel is white to grayish-white but appears slightly yellow because it is translucent. The underlying dentin is yellowish, giving the yellow tint to enamel.

Enamel ranges in thickness from a knifelike edge at its cervical margin to about a 2.5-mm maximum thickness over the occlusal or incisal surface.

■ Clinical Comment

Although enamel is the hardest tissue in the human body, it is permeable to some fluids, bacteria, and bacterial products of the oral cavity. Cracks, clefts, and microscopic spaces in and between rods and crystals allow penetration.

■ Rod Structure

Enamel is composed of rods that extend from their site of origin, at the dentinoenamel junction, to the enamel outer surface (Figure 7.1). Each rod is formed by ameloblasts; in fact, four ameloblasts form a part of each rod (Figure 7.2).

A rod is **keyhole-** or racquet-shaped with a head and a tail, as can be seen in Figure 7.2. The head of the rod is the broadest part, measuring 5 μ wide, and the elongated thinner portion, or tail, is about 1 μ wide. The rod is 9 μ long. The enamel rod is therefore about the same size as a red blood cell (Figure 7.3).

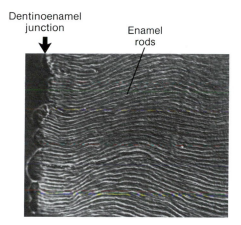

Figure 7.1 *Enamel rods appear wavy in this section as they extend from the dentinoenamel junction (DEJ) on the right to the enamel surface. This picture is possible because the section is etched and viewed on a scanning electron microscope.*

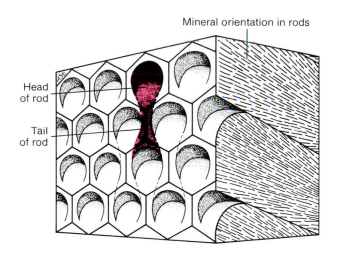

Figure 7.2 *This diagram shows the outline of six-sided ameloblasts overlying the keyhole-shaped enamel rods. Observe that parts of four cells form each enamel rod. On the side of the model can be seen the crystal orientation of the three rods.*

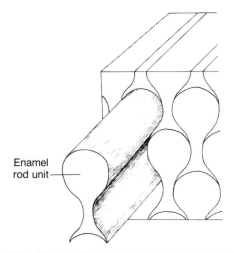

Figure 7.3 *One rod is pulled out to illustrate how individual enamel rods interdigitate with their neighbors.*

Each rod is filled with crystals. Those in the head follow the long axis of the rod, and those in the tail follow the direction of its long axis (Figure 7.4). The right half of Figure 7.4 indicates how the mineral is oriented during development in the rod, which forms the head and tail seen on the left. The architecture of the mineral orientation is complex, especially when viewed in any direction other than cross section (Figure 7.5).

Rods are formed nearly perpendicular to the dentino-enamel junction and curve slightly toward the cusp tip. This unique rod arrangement also undulates throughout the enamel to the surface. Each rod interdigitates with its neighbor, the head of one nestling against the neck of the rods to its left or right (see Figure 7.3). The rods run almost perpendicular to the enamel surface at the cervical region but are gnarled and intertwine near the cusp tips (Figure

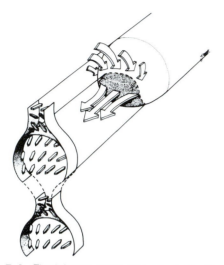

Figure 7.4   *The left side of the diagram shows the orientation of the crystals in the forming rod head and tail. The right shows how the forming crystals pack in the rod from the cell complex.*

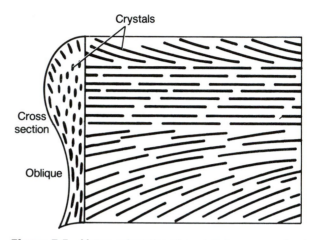

Figure 7.5   *Mature orientation of crystals in an enamel rod.*

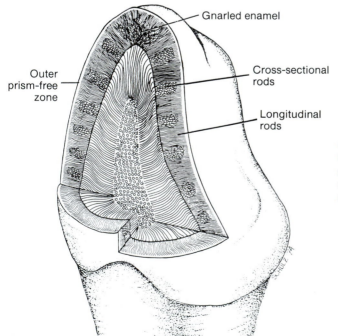

Figure 7.6   *Enamel rod orientation in enamel. At the cusp tips, enamel rods are gnarled. In the long axis of the crown, groups of enamel rods are bent at a different axis than adjacent groups. At the surface of the enamel the prisms are indistinct and oriented perpendicular to the surface.*

7.6). Each rod's surface is known as the rod sheath and its center is the core. The rod sheath contains slightly more organic matter than the rod core (Figure 7.7).

Groups of rods bend to the right or left at a slightly different angle than do the adjacent group of rods, as seen in the model (see Figure 7.6). It is believed that this feature provides enamel with strength for mastication and biting. When light is projected on the surface of a thin slab of enamel, light and dark bands appear. These bands are seen because the light transmits down the long axis of one group of rods and not along the adjacent group. One group of rods are bent at an angle as seen by the angle of light projected through this specimen (Figure 7.8). These bands are named **Hunter-Schreger bands** after the dental scientist who first noted this light and dark band phenomenon in enamel. This pattern is repeated from the cervical to the incisal areas when viewed along the long axis of the tooth. Hunter-Schreger bands extend through about one-half the thickness of the enamel as can be observed in the diagram (see Figure 7.6) and the tooth section (Figure 7.8).

■ *Clinical Comment*

The rods that form enamel are woven during formation into a mass that resists an average masticatory impact of 20 to 30 pounds per tooth. Enamel is thickest over the areas of greatest impact.

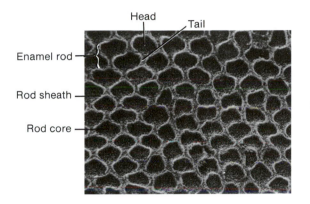

Figure 7.7 *Parallel enamel rods in cross section. Observe the rod head, tail, core, and sheath.*

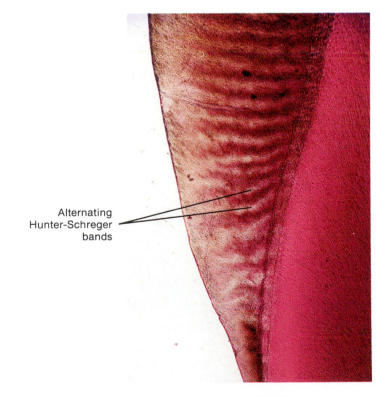

Figure 7.8 *A photomicrograph of enamel, taken by reflected light to illustrate the alternating light and dark Hunter-Schreger bands (S).*

■ Incremental Lines

The incremental line system, or lines of **Retzius,** in enamel is the rhythmic recurrent deposition by an appositional pattern. The enamel matrix then mineralizes, providing dark lines that indicate the growth lines (Figure 7.9). In cross section of the crown, these lines appear as concentric rings. At these lines, it is believed both that fewer crystals exist and that the enamel rods may bend slightly or constrict. Because many ameloblasts simultaneously deposit enamel rods, hypocalcified lines appear where the ameloblasts hesitate during enamel production. The resultant lines establish each successive contour of enamel matrix during its deposition. Therefore, small air spaces may develop and provide the dark lines noted. One of the early investigators who described these lines was **Retzius,** after whom these incremental lines were named the **striae of Retzius.**

Part of the enamel of deciduous teeth is formed both before and after birth. This abrupt change in environment and nutrition at birth is recorded in the enamel as a more pronounced **incremental line,** termed the **neonatal line** (Figure 7.9). The enamel matrix internal to this line represents the enamel formed before birth, and the enamel matrix external to it is formed after birth. Enamel formed before birth is whiter and contains fewer defects than that formed after birth. The neonatal line is an accentuated line, believed due to birth, and is seen in all teeth that were forming at birth (Figure 7.9). Therefore, most primary teeth and the permanent central incisors have incremental lines.

■ Clinical Comment

Enamel is composed of the same mineral found in dentin, bone, and cementum. Unlike with bone and cementum, this mineral is not replaced once it is deposited in enamel.

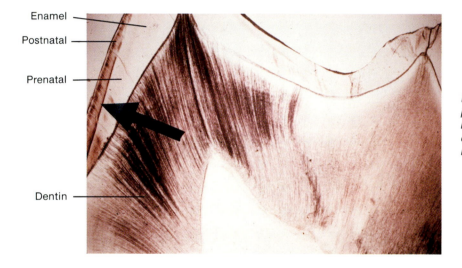

Figure 7.9 *Photomicrograph of a primary tooth section by transmitted light, illustrating structures found in enamel and dentin. Arrows indicates neonatal line.*

Figure 7.10 *A photomicrograph of enamel and dentin, taken by transmitted light to illustrate the neonatal line. Prenatal enamel is that portion of the enamel formed before birth, and postnatal enamel is formed after birth. The neonatal line is formed by the coalescence of the pre- and postnatally formed enamel.*

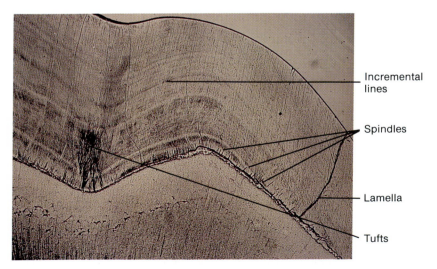

■ *Enamel Lamellae*

Enamel lamellae are visible cracks on the surface of enamel (Figure 7.10 and 7.11*A*). Lamellae extend for varying depths from the enamel surface toward the dentinoenamel junction. Some lamellae develop during enamel formation and some are created during tooth function. During formation of enamel rods and mineralization, spaces between rods or rod groups develop. These spaces are filled with organic material (protein) that persists as a lamella. Cracks may also appear in enamel. Because enamel is a highly mineralized tissue, stress from breathing cold air or drinking cold beverages may cause small checks to occur in enamel, especially enamel weakened by underlying caries. Lamellae are not tubular defects but appear more leaflike, extending around the crown (Figure 7.11*B*). Lamellae are important as a pathway through enamel and function as a possible avenue for dental caries.

■ *Enamel Tufts*

Enamel tufts are another defect in enamel filled with organic material. They arise from the dentinoenamel junction and are at right angles to it. They extend possibly one fifth to one tenth of the distance from the junction to the surface of the tooth (see Figure 7.9). Tufts are formed between enamel rod groups, which are oriented in different directions at the dentinoenamel junction. Spaces develop between adjacent groups of rods which are filled with organic material. These spaces are tuftlike and contain the organic material enamelin (Figure 7.12). When caries has spread from the tooth's surface to near the dentinoenamel junction, these hypocalcified tufts cause a lateral spread along this junction. The interface of the junction of dentin and enamel is scalloped, and often tufts arise from these scalloped peaks (Figure 7.12).

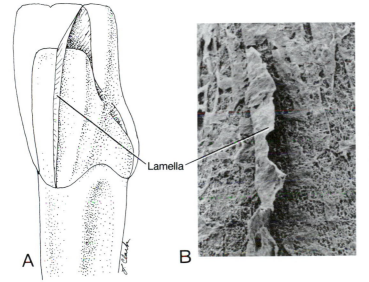

Lamella

A   B

Figure 7.11   (A) *Enamel lamellae penetrating enamel. These lamellae may extend from the incisal to the cervical areas. (B) Scanning electron micrograph of enamel lamellae.*

Figure 7.12 *Scanning electron micrograph of enamel tufts seen as organic tracts that allow penetration of bacteria and bacterial products to the dentinoenamel junction.*

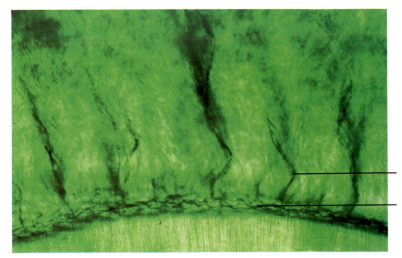

Enamel tufts

Dentinoenamel junction

■ *Enamel Spindles*

Spindles, which also arise from the dentinoenamel junction, are the extensions of dentinal tubules that penetrate the junction into enamel. Because the dentin forms before the enamel, the odontoblastic process occasionally penetrates the junction and then the enamel forms around it. Consequently, a small tubule, occasionally containing a process, is present in the enamel (Figure 7.13). These tubules are sometimes found singly or in groups and are shorter than tufts, only a few millimeters in length. The finger-like spindles appear quite different from the tufts.

■ *Surface Characteristics*

The enamel surface may be smooth or may have fine ridges. Such ridges result from the striae of Retzius terminating on the surface of the enamel (Figure 7.14). These surface manifestations, called **perikymata** or **imbrication lines,** are ridges produced by the ends of one group of rods accentuated over the space created before the next group becomes complete (Figure 7.15). This manifestation is particularly prominent on the facial surface of the teeth, near the cervical region. Another feature of the enamel near its surface is **prismless enamel,** measuring 20 to 40 μ thick. Most of the time prismless enamel is not accentuated but is more evident near the cervical region and in deciduous teeth (see Figure 7.6).

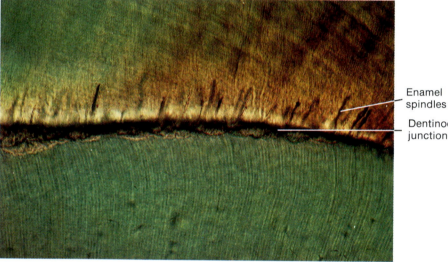

Enamel
spindles

Dentinoenamel
junction

Figure 7.13   *Enamel spindles at the dentinoenamel junction are extensions of dental tubules containing odontoblast processes in enamel.*

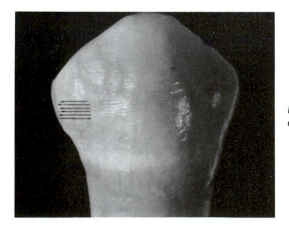

Figure 7.14   *Perikymata or imbrication lines on surface of enamel.*

■ Permeability

Enamel permeability is a feature of clinical importance. The passage of fluid, bacteria, and bacterial products through enamel is an important consideration in clinical therapy. Permeability of enamel is caused by several factors, some of which are evident as they relate to decomposition of the tooth by caries. Fine particles enter enamel through several pathways, namely, lamellae, microlamellae, tufts, and spindles. All except microlamella have been previously defined. **Microlamellae** are spaces between groups of rods, between individual rods, and through crystal spaces within rods. All of these structures influence the permeability of enamel.

■ Etching

The surface of enamel may be altered by etching with dilute acids, such as citric acid. This dilute acid selectively etches the ends of the enamel rods to allow adherence of a plastic sealant (Figure 7.16). The purpose of this procedure is to prevent caries, usually on the occlusal surface.

■ Clinical Comment

Some etched areas of enamel can be remineralized by solutions of sodium or stannous fluoride. Tests show the fluoride ion penetrates the porous demineralized enamel. Low levels of fluoride stimulate remineralization.

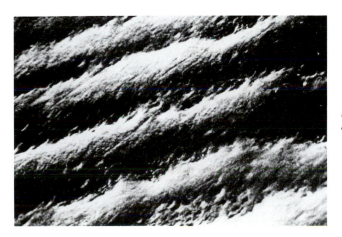

Figure 7.15 *Scanning electron micrograph of perikymata as seen in Figure 7.14 but at higher magnification.*

Rod head

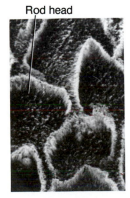

Figure 7.16 *Acid-etched enamel with rod head dissolved.*

■ Self-Evaluation Questions

1. Describe the shape and size of enamel rods.
2. Define Hunter-Schreger bands.
3. Define striae of Retzius. What is another name?
4. Describe gnarled enamel. Where is it located?
5. What are perikymata or imbrication lines?
6. What are the location and importance of tufts?
7. Define and give the cause of neonatal lines.
8. What is prismless enamel?
9. What is the inorganic component of enamel, dentin, and bone?
10. What is the organic component of enamel?

■ Acknowledgments

Figures 7.1 to 7.3, 7.5 to 7.7, and 7.11 to 7.16 kindly provided by Dr. J.W. Simmelink, Professor of Oral Biology, School of Dentistry, Case Western Reserve University, Cleveland, Ohio. These figures are reprinted from Histology of Enamel, in Avery, J.K., ed. *Oral Development and Histology,* Toronto: B.C. Decker, 1988.

■ Suggested Reading

Nylen, M.U., and Termine, J.D., eds. Tooth enamel III: Its development, structure, and composition. J. Dent. Res. 1979; 58(B):675.

Scott, D.B., Simmelink, J.W., and Nygaard, V.K. Structural aspects of dental caries. J. Dent. Res. 1974; 53:165.

Simmelink, J.W., and Nygaard, V.K. Ultrastructure of striations in carious human enamel. Caries Res. 1982; 16:179.

Stack, M.V., and Fearnhead, R.W., eds. Tooth enamel: Its composition, properties and fundamental structure. Bristol, UK: John Wright & Sons, 1965.

Dentin

■ Overview

This chapter focuses on dentin, which constitutes the entire body of the tooth, including the root, except for the covering by cementum, and constitutes much of the crown underlying the enamel. Dentin, like bone, is composed of an organic matrix of collagen fibers and the mineral hydroxyapatite. It is classified as primary, secondary, or tertiary on the basis of the time of its development and the histologic appearance of the tissue. Primary dentin, the first type discussed, is the major component of the crown and root, and consists of mantle dentin along the dentinoenamel junction. The collagen fibers in this narrow 150-micron-wide zone are larger than those of the remaining dentin, and this dentin is nearly defect-free. Mantle dentin is separated from the remainder of the primary dentin by the globular dentin. Globular dentin is a defect in mineralization that results in spaces appearing between globules. Primary dentin is formed until the tooth has reached occlusion and is functioning; then dentinogenesis slows and a secondary dentin is formed. The name secondary dentin is used to distinguish dentin formed much more slowly than the earlier-formed primary dentin. Usually there is little difference in appearance of dentin at the point of change from primary to secondary. A third type of dentin is formed in response to disease or trauma, called tertiary or reparative dentin. Bordering the pulp is a **predentin** zone, which is noncalcified and is the earliest-formed zone of dentoid composed of collagen fibers. It calcifies within 24 hours, as another band of predentin is forming pulpward.

In addition to classifying dentin, this chapter describes properties and characteristics of dentin. Like bone cells, the cells that form dentin lie on the surface of the hard tissue, but unlike bone the processes of the dentin-forming cells penetrate the dentin and lie within tubules. Dentin, like bone, is deposited by appositional growth and is characterized by **incremental lines,** as are bone, cementum and enamel. Root dentin contains a **granular layer** of dentin located along the root's surface. Loss of the odontoblastic process and fluid in the tubule result in **dead tracts,** and the occludent mineral obliterating the tubules results in **sclerotic dentin.**

■ Physical Properties

Dentin, which forms the bulk of the tooth, is yellowish in contrast to the whiter enamel. It appears darker if a root canal has been performed. Dentin is composed of 70 percent inorganic hydroxyapatite crystals, 20 percent organic collagen fibers along with small amounts of other proteins, and 10 percent water by weight. With 20 percent less mineral than enamel, it is softer, although it is slightly harder than bone or cementum. Therefore, it is radiographically more radiolucent than enamel but much more radiopaque than the pulp. Dentin is resilient or slightly elastic, which allows the impact of mastication to occur without fracturing the brittle overlying enamel. This resilience is due, in part, to the presence of tubules throughout the matrix which extend from the dentinoenamel junction to the pulp.

■ Clinical Comment

Metallic restorations such as gold and silver amalgam are excellent thermal conductors. Therefore, it is appropriate to place a low-conducting cement base under these restorations.

■ Dentin Classification

Dentin is composed of **primary dentin,** constituting most of the tooth; **secondary dentin,** a zone of variable thickness adjacent to the pulp; and **tertiary** or **reparative dentin,** formed in response to disease or trauma to the pulp. Examples of these classifications are shown in Figure 8.1.

Primary Dentin

Primary dentin is composed peripherally of a thin layer, approximately 150 μm thick, of **mantle dentin.** Mantle dentin is the initial dentin formed, and its collagen fibers are larger, 0.1 to 0.2 μm in diameter, in contrast to the remaining dentinal matrix, which is 50 to 200 nm. Mantle dentin is slightly less mineralized and contains fewer defects than the remainder of the primary dentin.

Adjacent to this band of primary dentin is a zone of **interglobular dentin,** better termed **globular dentin.** Globular dentin is seen in the crown adjacent to the dentinoenamel junction, and it may extend into the root. This zone of dentinal matrix was not mineralized properly, and areas of globular calciforites did not fuse correctly. This

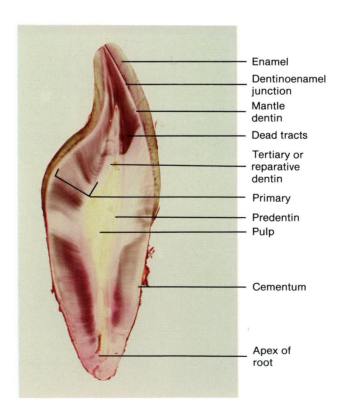

Enamel

Dentinoenamel junction

Mantle dentin

Dead tracts

Tertiary or reparative dentin

Primary

Predentin

Pulp

Cementum

Apex of root

Figure 8.1   Dentin terminology: location and distribution of various types of dentin.

dentin contains fewer mineralized areas between the globules, which are termed interglobular spaces (Figure 8.2). This diagram shows examples of various structures found in dentin. Interglobular spaces are not true spaces, but hypomineralized areas between the calcified globules. The dentinal tubules run without interruption through this zone, indicating a defect in mineralization and not in matrix formation (Figure 8.3). Interglobular dentin is especially noticeable with vitamin D deficiency, which affects mineral-

ization of teeth and bones. In the remaining 80 percent of primary dentin and, the collagen fibers are smaller and, more defects appear throughout this dentin than in mantle dentin. Primary dentin constitutes most of the dentin in both the crown and the root. It is characterized by the continuity of tubules from the dentinoenamel junction to the pulp and by incremental lines indicating a daily pattern of rhythmic deposition, of dentin of approximately 4 μm per day.

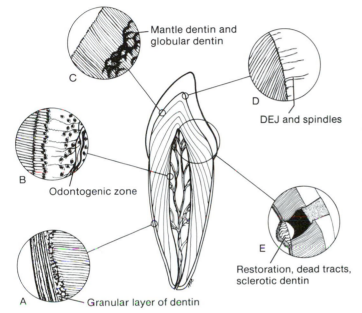

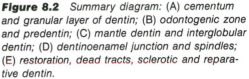

Figure 8.2 *Summary diagram: (A) cementum and granular layer of dentin; (B) odontogenic zone and predentin; (C) mantle dentin and interglobular dentin; (D) dentinoenamel junction and spindles; (E) restoration, dead tracts, sclerotic and reparative dentin.*

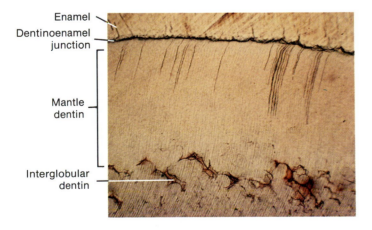

Figure 8.3 *Mantle dentin with interglobular spaces underneath and dentinoenamel junction above.*

Secondary Dentin

Secondary dentin is formed internal to the primary dentin of the crown and root. It develops after the crown has come into clinical function and the roots are nearly completed (Figure 8.4). This dentin is deposited more slowly than the primary dentin, and as a result, the incremental lines are only about 1.0 to 1.5 μm apart. Investigators theorize that after the crown comes into clinical function, the tooth signals the dentin to slow its rate of production. In this manner, the pulp is not obliterated by an excessive rate of dentin formation. The tubules of the primary and secondary dentin are generally continuous, unless the deposition of the secondary dentin is uneven. In molar teeth, for example, there is a greater deposit of secondary dentin on the roof and floor of the coronal pulp chamber than on the lateral walls. This leads to protection of the pulpal horns as aging occurs.

Tertiary or Reparative Dentin

Tertiary or reparative dentin results from pulpal stimulation and forms only at the site of odontoblastic activation. Whether due to attrition, abrasion, caries, or restorative procedures, this dentin is deposited underlying only those stimulated areas (Figures 8.5 and 8.6). It may be deposited rapidly, in which case the resulting dentin appears irregular with sparse and twisted tubules and possible cell inclusions (Figure 8.6*B* to *D*). Odontoblasts, fibroblasts, and blood cells have all been found in this type of dentin. In contrast, if it is formed slowly because of less extreme stimuli, the dentin appears more regular, much like primary or secondary dentin (Figure 8.6*A*). At times, this dentin resembles bone more than dentin and is termed **osteodentin** (Figure 8.6*C*), or it appears as a combination of several types (Figure 8.6*E*).

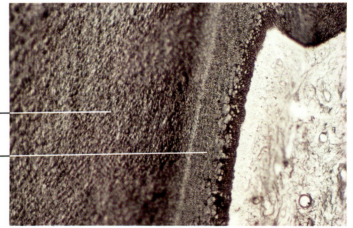

Figure 8.4 *Primary dentin* (left) *and secondary dentin* (right).

Primary dentin

Secondary dentin

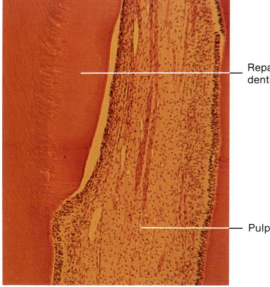

Reparative dentin

Pulp

Figure 8.5 *Reparative dentin formed in a localized area underlying a cavity. Note that tubules from the cavity floor lead to reparative dentin.*

■ *Predentin*

Predentin is that band of newly formed, and as yet un-mineralized, matrix of dentin located at the pulpal border of the dentin (Figure 8.7). Predentin is evidence that dentin forms in two stages—first, the organic matrix is deposited and, second, an inorganic mineral substance is added. The predentin zone may be 4 μm wide during early primary dentin formation but only 1.0 to 1.5 μm when secondary dentin forms. Mineralization of this dentin occurs at the predentin-dentin junction, and as the previous predentin becomes dentin, a new layer of predentin is formed.

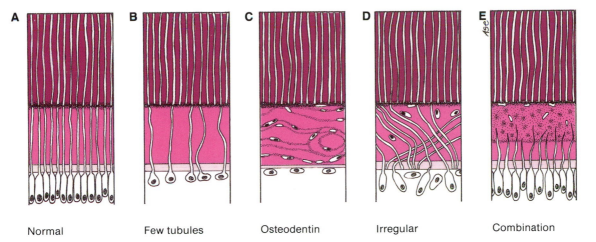

| Normal | Few tubules | Osteodentin | Irregular | Combination |

Figure 8.6 *Normal dentin (A) and reparative dentin (B to E). Reparative dentin contains fewer than normal tubules (B), or it includes cells within its matrix. (C) shows irregularly arranged tubules (D), or is a combination of different types (E).*

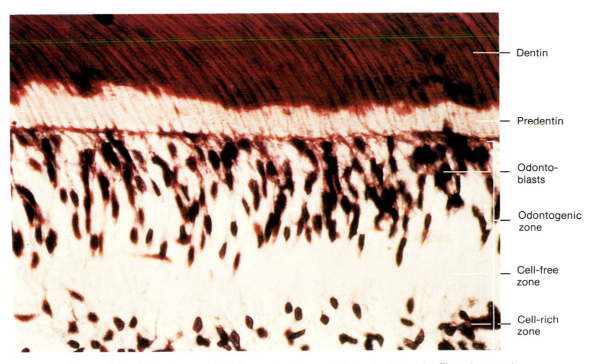

Dentin

Predentin

Odonto-blasts

Odontogenic zone

Cell-free zone

Cell-rich zone

Figure 8.7 *Photomicrograph of the predentin zone that borders the pulp. The odontogenic zone is seen below the predentin. This zone is composed of the odontoblasts, cell-free and cell-rich zones.*

■ Tubular and Intertubular Relations

Primary and Secondary Tubules

As dentin is formed by odontoblasts, space is provided for the ever-lengthening process of the odontoblast as it moves pulpward from the dentinoenamel junction to in front of the layer of predentin. The tubules normally begin perpendicular to the dentinoenamel and the dentinocemental junction to the pulp, forming an **S** curve (see Figure 8.1). These cells and their branching processes provide the vitality of the dentin (Figure 8.8). The ratio of the amount of surface area of the dentinoenamel junction to the pulpal surface is about 5 to 1. Therefore, the tubules are farther apart at the dentinoenamel junction than at the pulpal surface (Figure 8.8). In addition, they are smaller in diameter at the outer dentin (1 μm) than at the pulpal border (3 to 4 μm). The ratio of the number of tubules in the outer dentin to those in the pulpal zone is about 4 to 1. There are also more tubules in the crown than in the root, and 30,000 to 50,000 tubules per square millimeter are found near the pulp. Throughout dentin, the tubules exhibit lateral branches that arise at right angles to the main tubule. They are termed canaliculi; secondary, lateral branches; or microtubules (see Figure 8.8). These branches are less than a micrometer in diameter and arise more or less at right angles to the main tubule. Some of the canaliculi enter adjacent main tubules, and some appear to terminate in the intertubular matrix. They contain lateral branches of the main odontoblastic process.

Intratubular or Peritubular Dentin

The dentinal matrix that immediately surrounds the dentinal tubule is termed **intratubular** or **peritubular dentin** (Figure 8.9). Peritubular dentin is present throughout dentin, except in the tubules near the pulp. It is about 40 percent more highly calcified than the adjacent **intertubular dentin.** Since this hypermineralized collar of dentin surrounds the tubules, it has long been called peritubular dentin. However, because it is formed within and at the expense of the dentinal tubules, **intratubular dentin** is a more accurate term.

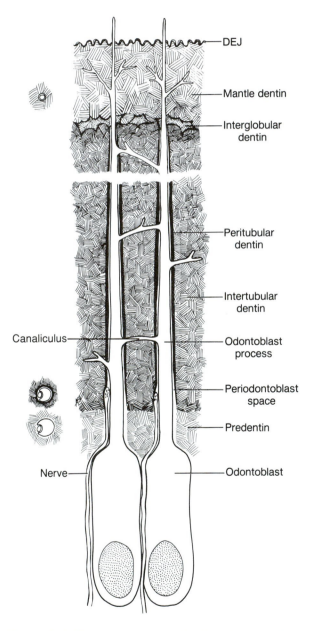

Figure 8.8   *The process of the odontoblast in its tubule extends throughout dentin into tubules in the inner enamel. Note the side branches of the processes in tubules, termed canaliculi. DEJ = dentinoenamel junction.*

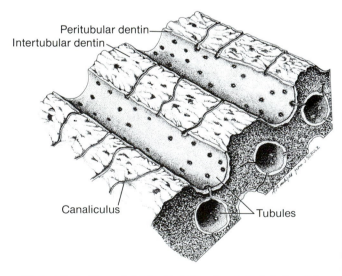

Figure 8.9   *View of dentinal tubules shows peritubular and intertubular dentin. Note the side branches of dentinal tubules.*

It is interesting to observe that intratubular dentin is missing from the dentinal tubules in interglobular dentin, indicating that this is a defect of mineralization. In some areas, the intratubular dentin completely obliterates the tubules—for example, near the dentinoenamel junction overlying the pulp horns and especially in the root. When the tubules are completely obliterated in an area of dentin, this is called **sclerotic dentin** or **transparent dentin** (Figure 8.10). The name is derived from the transparent nature of dentin, which manifests when the tubules are no longer present. Sclerotic dentin increases in amount with age and is believed to be a protective mechanism of the pulp, to decrease permeability, and to prevent irritation to the pulp in an area of overlying attrition, abrasion, fracture, or caries of the enamel.

Intertubular Dentin

The main body of dentin, known as intertubular dentin, is located between each dentinal tubule or zone of intratubular dentin. Intertubular dentin, like intratubular dentin, is composed of an organic matrix of type I collagen fibers and inorganic crystals of hydroxyapatite. It is, however, less highly mineralized and, unlike intratubular dentin, changes little throughout life. The collagen fibers of the matrix form a meshwork oriented in a near perpendicular direction to the intratubular dentin. They exhibit a typical 640 Å cross banding.

■ *Clinical Comment*

Dentin is a permeable hard tissue with tubules leading from the dentinoenamel junction to the pulp. Effective sealing of dentinal tubules is a requisite of restorative dentistry.

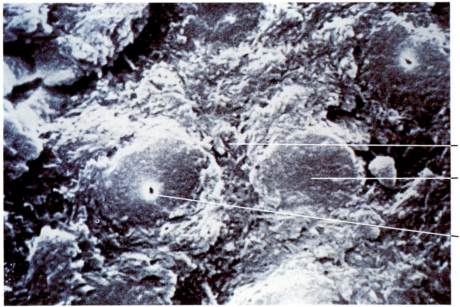

Intertubular dentin

Occluded tubules

Near-occluded tubule

Figure 8.10 *Scanning electron micrograph of sclerotic dentin tubules.*

■ *Incremental Lines*

All dentin is deposited incrementally, which means that as a certain amount of matrix is deposited daily, a hesitation in activity follows. This lack of formation results in lines known as **incremental lines, imbrication lines,** or **lines of von Ebner.** Although daily lines are difficult to distinguish, lines formed from increments deposited over several days (possibly five days), resulting in 20 μm, are known as von Ebner

lines (Figure 8.11). Analysis of soft x-ray films has shown these lines to represent hypocalcified bands. In the primary dentition and the first permanent molar teeth, in which dentin is formed partly before and after birth, the prenatal and postnatal dentin are separated by an accentuated contour line known as the **neonatal line** (Figure 8.12). This reflects the abrupt change in environment that occurs at or near birth.

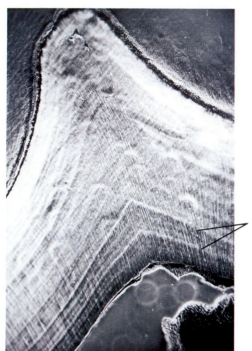

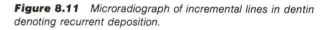
Incremental
lines

Figure 8.11   *Microradiograph of incremental lines in dentin denoting recurrent deposition.*

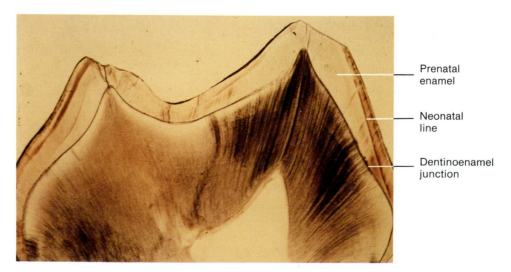

Prenatal
enamel

Neonatal
line

Dentinoenamel
junction

Figure 8.12   *The neonatal line is easily seen in enamel because of the color change in the postnatal enamel. In dentin it appears as an accentuated incremental line visible under the microscope.*

■ Granular Layer

When ground sections of root dentin are studied under transmitted light, there is a granular zone underlying the cementum covering the root. Known as **Tomes' granular layer** (Figure 8.13), this zone increases slightly in width, proceeding from the cementoenamel junction to the root apex. The zone is believed due to a coalescing and looping of the terminal portions of the dentinal tubules. It is possible that the odontoblast is initially disoriented, turns until oriented at right angles to the root sheath, and then proceeds in an orderly fashion, leaving a straight tubule behind (Figure 8.14).

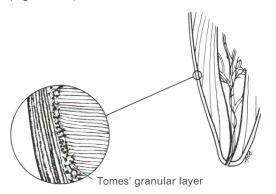

Tomes' granular layer

Figure 8.13 *Appearance and location of granular layer of dentin along the cementodentinal junction of the root.*

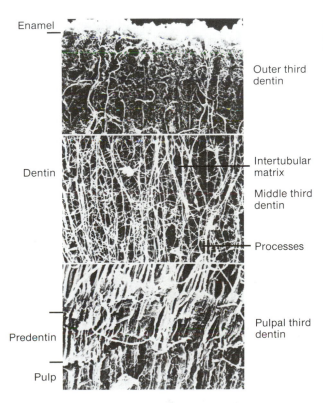

Enamel

Dentin

Predentin

Pulp

Outer third dentin

Intertubular matrix

Middle third dentin

Processes

Pulpal third dentin

Figure 8.15 *Photograph of odontoblasts (bottom) with their processes intact and extending to the dentinoenamel junction (top). The peritubular or intertubular dentin matrix has been removed.*

■ Odontoblastic Cell Processes

The odontoblastic cell processes are the cytoplasmic extensions of the odontoblast, which exists in the peripheral pulp. There is some disagreement as to whether these processes extend through the entire thickness of dentin. This difference of opinion is due, in part, to the difficulty of preserving and visualizing these processes. Recently, improved techniques of immunofluorescent labeling, freeze fracture, and polymer replacement have revealed that these structures extend to the dentinoenamel junction (Figure 8.15). In some instances, they also extend into the enamel for a short distance as enamel spindles (Figure 8.16). The odontoblastic processes are largest in diameter

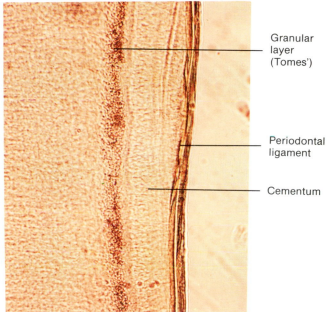

Granular layer (Tomes')

Periodontal ligament

Cementum

Figure 8.14 *Histologic appearance of granular layer of dentin (center) and cementum (near right). PDL = periodontal ligament (far right).*

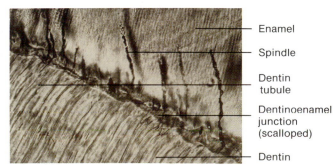

Enamel

Spindle

Dentin tubule

Dentinoenamel junction (scalloped)

Dentin

Figure 8.16 *Spindles, which are extensions of dentinal tubules, pass across the dentinoenamel junction into the inner enamel.*

near the pulp (3 to 4 μm) and taper to 1 μm near the dentinoenamel junction. These processes divide near the dentinoenamel junction to end in several branched processes (Figure 8.17). Periodically along the odontoblastic processes, lateral branches arise at near right angles to the main odontoblastic process and extend into the intertubular dentin or into the adjacent tubules (see Figure 8.15). The odontoblastic process contains microtubules, small filaments, occasional mitochondria, and microvessicles. This is indicative of the protein-secreting nature of the odontoblast. Nerve terminals can also be seen in the dentinal tubule, in the region of the predentin and adjacent dentin. These are described in Chapter 9 on pulp.

Loss of the odontoblastic process usually results in the appearance of **dead tracts** in dentin. In the dentin underlying an area of attrition or a carious lesion, the odontoblasts may die and disintegrate, producing a band of dead tracts in the dentin. When this condition exists, the tubules become air filled. When a ground section is made, air becomes incorporated, resulting in a black appearance of these tubules (Figure 8.18).

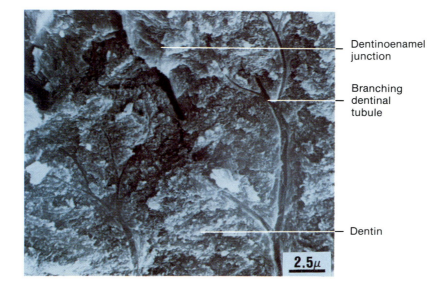

— Dentinoenamel junction

— Branching dentinal tubule

— Dentin

2.5μ

Figure 8.17 *Observe the branching of the dentinal tubules near the dentinoenamel junction in this scanning electron micrograph.*

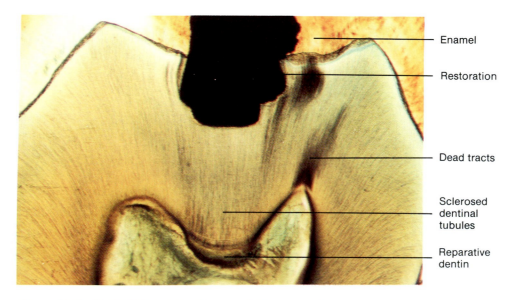

— Enamel

— Restoration

— Dead tracts

— Sclerosed dentinal tubules

— Reparative dentin

Figure 8.18 *Dead tracts or open tubules underlie a restoration and are often associated with sclerosed dentinal tubules.*

■ *Dentinoenamel Junction*

The junction between the dentin and enamel is scalloped or has ridges that enhance the contact of the two. This is apparent only at high magnification, as seen in Figure 8.16. Scalloping has been reported greatest in the area of cusps where the incisal or occlusal trauma is intense. The dentinoenamel junction is characterized by several features other than scalloping. Several features are noted in the area of the dentinoenamel junction: (1) scalloping, (2) the appearance of spindles, and (3) the branching of the dentinal tubules. All of these are noted in Figures 8.16 and 8.17.

■ *Clinical Comment*

Dentin is a vital tissue containing living cell processes. Because this tissue permeates the tooth so completely in tubules and branching canaliculi, it is impossible to touch a cavity preparation with an explorer without producing pain.

■ *Permeability*

The outer surface of dentin is approximately 5 times larger than the inner surface. Since the tubule diameter is only 1 μm near the dentinoenamel junction, the tubules are farthest apart at this junction. However, they are much closer at the pulpal interface, since both the tubules are larger (3 to 4 μm) and the predentinal surface is smaller than the dentoenamel junction (see Figure 8.19). The tubules are consequently cone-shaped and permit increased permeability as the surface of the tubule enlarges with etching or dental caries. The system of branching tubules allows the permeability to increase further. One feature that works against this fluid flow through dentin is the higher osmotic pressure of the pulp as opposed to the dentinoenamel junction. Fluid is constantly being forced outward by this increased pressure of the pulp. Therefore, when a dentinal tubule is cut, a small vesicle of fluid usually appears on the cut surface. Against this flow, it has been found that minute particles such as bacteria or bacterial products can percolate down the dentinal tubules into the pulp. Again, the loss of the odontoblastic process which leads to the development of a dead tract results in increased permeability. For these reasons, the permeability factor is a major consideration in the cleansing of the cavity and the placement of a cavity liner to prevent microleakage. Note in Figure 8.19 that caries bacteria (the dotted area) find the shortest distance to the pulp along the dentinal tubules. Note location in the pulp of reparative dentin to the cavity.

■ *Repair Process*

Dentin is laid down throughout life. Pathologic effects of dental caries, attrition, abrasion, and the cutting of dentin cause changes in dentin. These are described as dead tracts, sclerosis, and tertiary or reparative dentin. The formation of dentin by increased dentinogenic activity underlying an area of injured odontoblastic processes is described as dentinal repair. Although the mechanisms underlying these processes are still not clear, the histologic changes following dentinal irritation are basically understood. Note that in the area underlying bacterial invasion, in Figure 8.19, the reparative dentin is thickest. The vitality of dentin is perhaps the most significant difference between this tissue and enamel, but future treatment of this tissue presents the ultimate challenge.

■ *Clinical Comment*

Irritation of dentin causes walling off of the pulp by mineral blocking of tubules and the addition of reparative dentin.

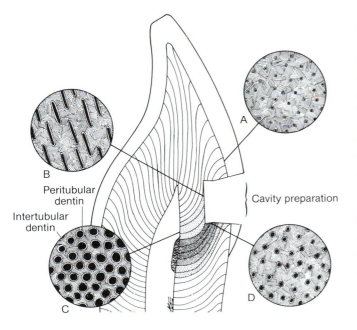

Figure 8.19 *Location and size of dentinal tubules at the dentinoenamel junction (A) and pulp (C). Relationship between the tubule in the cavity floor (B and D) and the pathway of caries through dentin. Compare the size of the tubules at the pulp (C) to the floor of the cavity (B and D) and the DEJ at (A).*

B
Peritubular dentin
Intertubular dentin
Cavity preparation
C
D

Sacramento City College Library

■ Self-Evaluation Questions

1. Name the type of dentin that composes the major portion of the crown and root.
2. Name the newly formed zone of collagen matrix that borders the pulp.
3. Which vitamin affects calcification of dentin and bone?
4. Describe the location of peritubular dentin. Is it more or less calcified than intertubular dentin?
5. Describe the location of the granular layer of Tomes.
6. What is the name for the extension of the odontoblast into enamel?
7. Compare the permeability of enamel and dentin.
8. Why is dentin considered a vital tissue?
9. Describe the location of mantle dentin and its characteristics.
10. Compare a zone of dead tracts to sclerotic dentin.

■ Acknowledgments

Figures 8.1 to 8.3 and 8.,10 to 8.19 are reprinted from Chapter 12, Histology of Dentin, in Avery, J.K., ed., *Oral Development and Histology,* Toronto, B.C. Decker, 1988. Figure 8.4, 8.6, 8.8, and 8.9 are reprinted from Chapter 4, Dentin, in Bhaskar, S.N., ed., *Orban's Oral Histology and Embryology,* St. Louis, C.V. Mosby, 1980. Figure 8.10 is reprinted by courtesy of Martin Branstrom, D.D.S. Figure 8.15 is reproduced by courtesy of Takahide Gunji, D.D.S.

■ Suggested Reading

Bergenholtz, G., Cox, C.F., Loesche, W.J., and Syed, S.A. Leakage around dental restorations and its effect on dental pulp. Pathology 1982; 11:439.

Mjor, I.A. Microradiography of human coronal dentin. Arch. Oral Biol. 1966; 11:225.

Szabo J., Trombitas, K., and Szabo I. The odontoblast process branches. Arch. Oral Biol. 1984; 26:331.

Trowbridge, H.O., Franks, M., Korostoffs, E., and Emling, R. Response to thermal stimulation in human teeth. J. Endocrinol. 1980; 6:40.

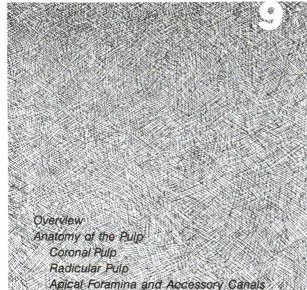

Dental Pulp

■ Overview

The dental pulp of each tooth has both a coronal, or crown, and a radicular, or root, element. It contains connective tissue, blood vessels, nerves, cells such as odontoblasts and fibroblasts, and various cells associated with the blood vessels and nerves. The connective tissue is delicate and the vessel walls are thin, since the pulp is entirely enclosed in a mantle of dentin. The pulp opens into the periodontium at the apical canal, at which point the characteristics of the tissue change. At the apex, accessory apical canals may be present.

Pulp has a central zone and a peripheral zone, which are observed both coronally and radicularly. The central zone contains the large arteries, veins, and nerve trunks that enter the apical canal and proceed to the coronal pulp chamber. Fibroblasts are the predominant pulp cell, existing in an intercellular substance of glycoaminoglycans and collagen fibers. The periphery is characterized by an odontogenic zone consisting of odontoblasts and cell-free and cell-rich zones. Adjacent to the cell-rich zone is a parietal layer of nerves.

Odontoblasts form dentin throughout life, which causes the pulp to become smaller with time. Pulpal vessels are thin-walled in the periphery, and the larger ones with muscles under sympathetic neural control are in the central pulp. There are several theories regarding pain conduction through dentin. However, the hydrodynamic theory is the most practical. It implies that dentin stimulation causes the odontoblasts and their processes to move into contact with nerve endings in the predentin and pulp. This results in mechanoreceptors receiving the impulses that conduct a pain response to the central nervous system.

Pulp has several functions, including initiative, formative, protective, nutritive, and reparative. The various protective functions are important clinical features.

The pulp may regress and contain diffuse areas or bundles of collagen fibers or true or false pulp stones. These pulp stones may be free, attached, or embedded in the dentin. Pulp may also contain diffuse calcifications.

■ Anatomy of the Pulp

The dental pulp consists of soft connective, vascular, lymphatic, and nervous tissue that occupies the center of each tooth. Humans have a total of 52 pulp organs, 20 primary and 32 permanent in each respective dentition (Figure 9.1). All pulp has similar morphologic characteristics, such as a soft gelatinous consistency which resides in a chamber surrounded by dentin containing the peripheral extensions of the formative cells. The total pulp volume for the permanent teeth is approximately 0.38 ml, and the mean volume of a single area of adult human pulp of 0.2 ml. The pulp of molar teeth is approximately four times larger than that of incisors (see Figure 9.1).

Coronal Pulp

There are two types of pulp: coronal and radicular, as seen in Figure 9.2. The **coronal pulp** occupies the crown of the tooth and resembles the crown shape at the outer surface of dentin in a young person. The pulp has six surfaces: the occlusal, mesial, distal, buccal, and lingual surfaces and the floor. There are also pulp horns, which are protrusions of the coronal pulp that extend into the cusps of teeth. The number of pulp horns, therefore, depends on the number of cusps (see Figure 9.1). At the cervical region, the coronal pulp joins the root. With age, the coronal pulp decreases in size owing to continued dentin formation (Figure 9.2*A-D).

Radicular Pulp

Pulpal root canals extend from the cervical region to the apex of the root. The **radicular pulp** of the anterior teeth is singular, whereas the posterior teeth have multiple pulps. Radicular pulp is tapered and conical and, like coronal pulp, becomes smaller with age owing to continued dentinogenesis (Figure 9.3). The apical canal may become further narrowed by cementum formation.

■ Clinical Comment

Knowledge of the pulp chamber shape and the extension of the pulp horns into the overlying cusps is most important to operative dentistry. Pulp horns can present a potential problem in pulp exposure.

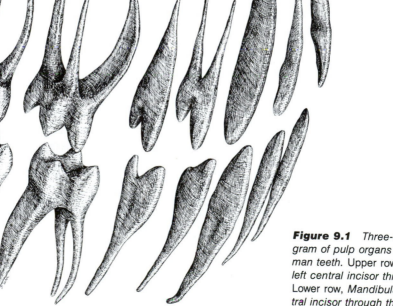

Figure 9.1 *Three-dimensional diagram of pulp organs of permanent human teeth. Upper row, Maxillary arch; left central incisor through third molar. Lower row, Mandibular arch; left central incisor through third molar.*

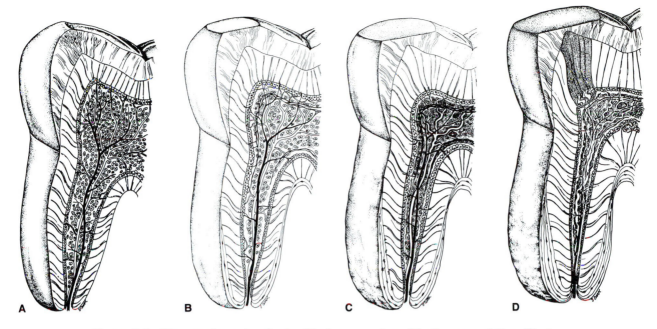

Figure 9.2 *Diagram of a series of pulps (A) at a young stage, (B) after some attrition, (C) at middle age, and (D) at old age. Note the decrease in the size of pulp and the alteration of dentin under the attrition zone.*

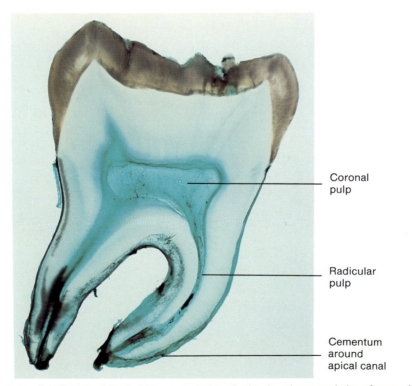

Coronal pulp

Radicular pulp

Cementum around apical canal

Figure 9.3 *Calcified section of older permanent tooth showing decreased size of coronal and radicular pulp.*

Apical Foramina and Accessory Canals

An **apical foramen** is the pulpal opening to the periodontium. This opening varies in size from 0.3 to 0.6 mm, being slightly larger in the maxillary than in the mandibular teeth. The apical foramen generally is centrally located in the newly formed root apex but becomes more eccentrically located with age (Figure 9.3). If several apical canals exist, the larger is designated the apical foramen and the more lateral ones are called accessory canals (Figure 9.4). Accessory canals may result from the presence of blood vessels obstructing dentin formation or the lack of a root sheath needed to induce early root formation. The incidence of accessory canals is said to be about 33 percent in the permanent teeth. Accessory canals are located on the lateral sides of the apical region and may also be found in the bifurcation area of multirooted teeth. Clinically, accessory canals are important because they represent contact of the pulp with the periodontal tissues. If inflammation of the pulp is present, it can spread to the periodontium or vice versa.

■ Clinical Comment

The presence of accessory pulp canals in an area where periodontal pathologic conditions exist may allow bacteria to spread into the pulp. If there is a pathologic condition of the pulp, on the other hand, it could be disseminated to the periodontium through such an accessory canal.

■ Histology of the Pulp

Centrally, the pulp is composed of large veins and arteries and nerve trunks and is surrounded by fibroblasts and collagen fibers embedded in an intercellular matrix (Figure 9.5,A). More peripherally, along the dentin in both the coronal and radicular pulp, are the formative cells of dentin and odontoblasts. The zone including and adjacent to these cells is known as the **odontogenic zone.** It is composed of the **odontoblasts,** the **cell-free zone,** and the **cell-rich zones,** (Figure 9.5,B). The cell-free zone is also known as the **zone of Weil** or **Weil's basal layer.** Adjacent to this zone is the cell-rich zone with high cell density, and adjacent to that is the parietal layer of nerves (Figure 9.5,B). Thus, the odontogenic zone is highly organized. It appears most notably in the coronal pulp and relates to the process of dentin formation, although the function of the cell-free and cell-rich zones in this process is still uncertain. In addition to the area of central and peripheral pulp is the region of the **pulp horns.** Here, the odontoblasts are crowded and appear palisaded in contrast to their appearance as a single layer of odontoblasts in most other areas of the pulp (Figure 9.6).

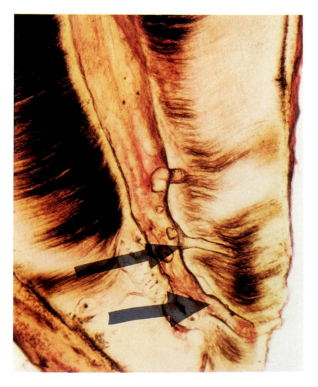

Figure 9.4 *Section of tooth apex illustrating an accessory canal at the upper arrow and the main apical canal at the lower arrow.*

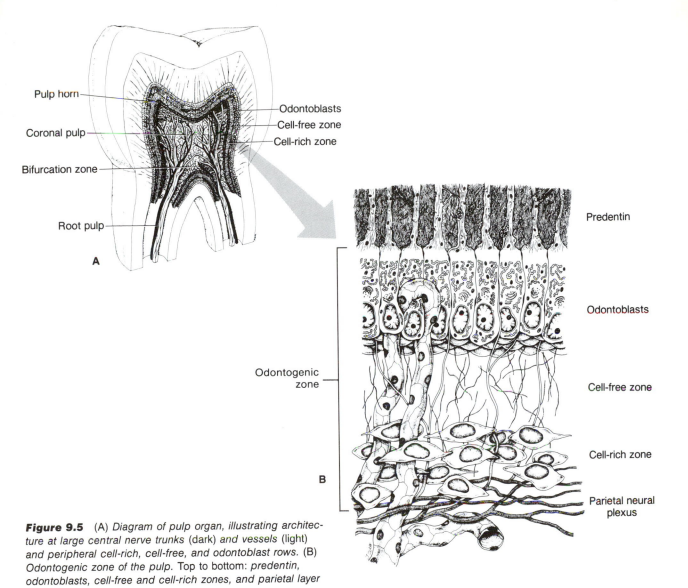

Pulp horn

Coronal pulp

Bifurcation zone

Root pulp

A

Odontoblasts
Cell-free zone
Cell-rich zone

Predentin

Odontoblasts

Cell-free zone

Cell-rich zone

Parietal neural plexus

Odontogenic zone

B

Figure 9.5 (A) *Diagram of pulp organ, illustrating architecture at large central nerve trunks* (dark) *and vessels* (light) *and peripheral cell-rich, cell-free, and odontoblast rows.* (B) *Odontogenic zone of the pulp.* Top to bottom: *predentin, odontoblasts, cell-free and cell-rich zones, and parietal layer of nerves.*

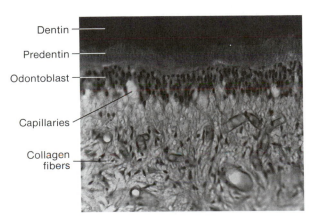

Dentin

Predentin

Odontoblast

Capillaries

Collagen fibers

Figure 9.6 *Photomicrograph of odontoblasts in the coronal area of the pulp organ. Notice pulpal capillaries among the cells.*

Odontoblastic Cells

Odontoblastic cells are small and round in their early differential stage and grow and become columnar as they become functional (Figure 9.7A to D). The odontoblasts are larger in the coronal pulp than in the root and appear columnar in the pulp horns (see Figure 9.6). These tall, columnar cells measure about 35 μm in length in the pulp horns, in contrast to cells in the radicular pulp, which are more cuboidal, and cells in the apical region, which appear flat.

The active cell has a large oval nucleus in its basal portion, and a Golgi's apparatus appears on the dentinal side of the nucleus. Abundant rough-surface endoplasmic reticulum and numerous mitochondria are scattered through the cell body (see Figure 9.9). The odontoblastic process arises from the odontoblast at the predentinal border where the cell constricts as the process enters the dentinal tubule (Figure 9.8). The process passes through the predentin with a few mitochondria and into the mineralized dentin, where it is devoid of major organelles, but contains filaments and microtubules through its length to the dentinoenamel junction. There has been some debate as to how far this process extends through the dentin. Recent information indicates it extends all the way to and, in some instances, through the dentinoenamel junction into enamel as spindles (Figure 9.8).

Three types of junctional complexes are found between adjacent odontoblasts: **tight (adhering), gap,** and **intermediate junctions** (Figure 9.10). Each has different functions. Adhering junctions, or **spot desmosomes,** are beltlike areas around these cells that possibly function in maintaining positional relationships between cells. This prevents substances in the pulp from leaking into the dentin. Gap junctions afford openings between odontoblasts for communication of electrical impulses and small molecules (Figures 9.10 and 9.11). In this manner, the odontoblasts can have synchronous activity with each other. If stimuli reach the odontoblasts, this information spreads throughout this cell layer by gap junctions.

Although odontoblasts are generally believed to live as long as the tooth is viable, inactivity and aging of the odontoblasts result in loss of organelles and a reduction in cell size.

■ Clinical Comment

The pulp horns recede with age. This is a protective measure performed by the pulp cells. Also, reparative dentin forms under cavity preparations. Cells in the pulp can be called upon to become new odontoblasts and form dentin at required sites.

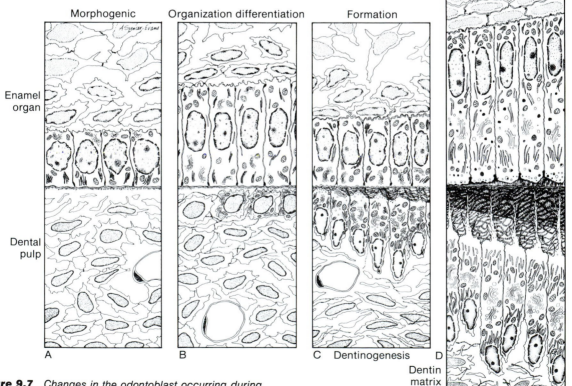

Figure 9.7 *Changes in the odontoblast occurring during differentiation. Observe changes in the preodontoblast in* A *to the functional odontoblast in* D.

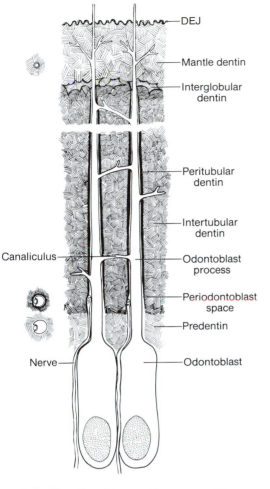

- DEJ
- Mantle dentin
- Interglobular dentin
- Peritubular dentin
- Intertubular dentin
- Odontoblast process
- Periodontoblast space
- Predentin
- Odontoblast

Canaliculus

Nerve

Figure 9.8 *The odontoblast and its process. The process extends through the entire thickness of dentin and into the inner enamel at the top of the picture. A cross section of the tubules is seen at the left.*

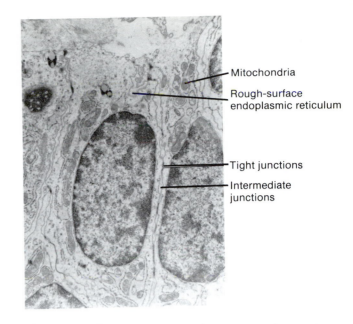

- Mitochondria
- Rough-surface endoplasmic reticulum
- Tight junctions
- Intermediate junctions

Figure 9.9 *Electron micrograph of tight, intermediate, and gap junctions which are found between odontoblasts. Cell organelles may also be seen in this photograph in the region of the nuclei.*

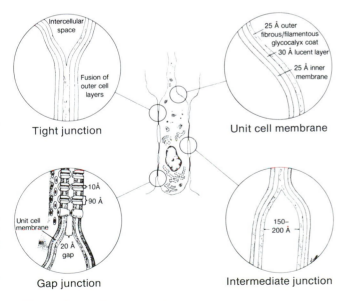

Intercellular space

Fusion of outer cell layers

Tight junction

25 Å outer fibrous/filamentous glycocalyx coat
30 Å lucent layer
25 Å inner membrane

Unit cell membrane

10 Å
90 Å

Unit cell membrane

20 Å gap

Gap junction

150–200 Å

Intermediate junction

Figure 9.10 *The types of junctional complexes between adjacent odontoblasts.*

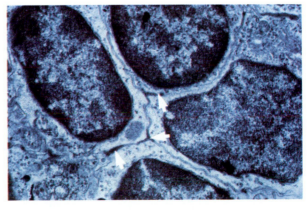

Figure 9.11 *Electron micrograph of the junction of four odontoblasts. Observe their nuclei and cell membranes meeting at thickened, dense staining zones where junctions are formed as indicated by the arrows. These dark zones are gap junctions that allow passage of small molecules between cells.*

Fibroblastic Cells

Fibroblasts are the most numerous cells seen throughout the pulp, although they exist in greater numbers in the cell-rich zone. Again, these cells are characterized by their functional state. In the young pulp, when they are producing collagen fibers and ground substance of the pulp, they are large cells, as can be observed in Figure 9.12. At that time, they have large multiple processes, with a centrally located oval nucleus, adjacent Golgi's apparatus, abundant rough-surface endoplasmic reticulum, and mitochondria (Figure 9.13). Later, in periods of less activity and aging, these cells appear smaller and spindle-shaped with few organelles.

Other Pulpal Cells

Nerve cells in the pulp include the **Schwann cells** (Figure 9.14). These cells form the myelin sheath of nerves and are associated with all the nerves of the pulp. In addition, **endothelial cells** lining the capillaries, veins, and arterioles of the pulp can be visualized (Figure 9.15). Accompanying most blood vessels are **pericytes** and numerous **undifferentiated cells** found in normal pulp. They function as a cell pool until called into action when a new odontoblast or fibroblast is needed. This may happen when there is a pulp exposure and reparative dentin needs to be formed. **Macrophages,** a normal constituent of the pulp, function in pulp maintenance, since there is a turnover of cells in the pulp (Figure 9.16). Lymphocytes are also found in the pulp-free spaces and probably function as an immune system of the pulp. **Erythrocytes, lymphocytes, leukocytes, eosinophils,** and **basophils** are found in blood vessels of the pulp.

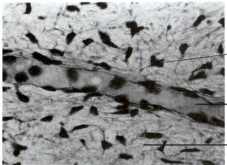

— Fibroblasts

— Blood vessel

— Collagen fibers

Figure 9.12 *Pulp fibroblasts, collagen fibers, and blood vessels in the pulp.*

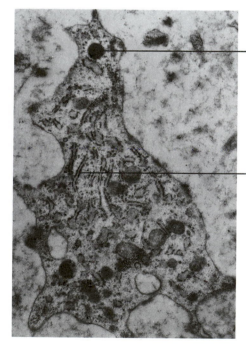

Mitochondria

Endoplasmic reticulum

Figure 9.13 *Electron micrograph of pulp fibroblasts showing organelles.*

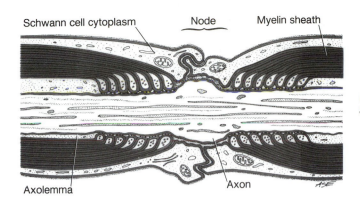

Schwann cell cytoplasm   Node   Myelin sheath

Axolemma   Axon

Figure 9.14 *Pulpal nerve axon surrounded by a Schwann cell.*

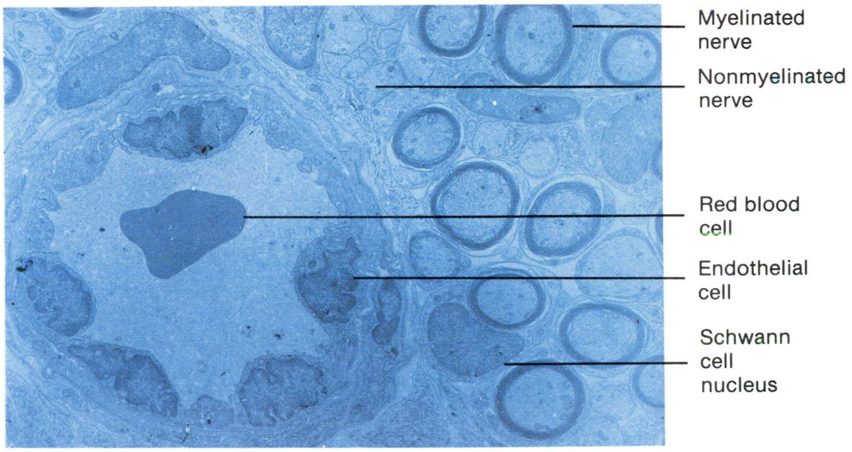

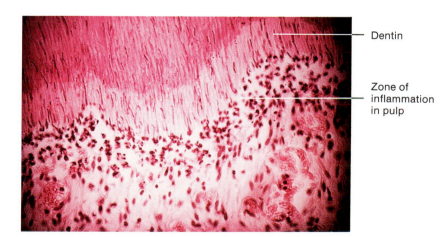

Myelinated nerve

Nonmyelinated nerve

Red blood cell

Endothelial cell

Schwann cell nucleus

Figure 9.15 *Electron micrograph of an arteriole in the central pulp. Its lumen is surrounded by endothelial cells and a layer of muscle cells. The endothelial cells comprise the intima and the muscle cells, the media. To the right are myelinated nerves; the large nuclei belong to Schwann cells.*

Dentin

Zone of inflammation in pulp

Figure 9.16 *Area underlying dentin with leukocytes and macrophages apparently responding to an irritant that resulted in inflammation.*

Fibers and Ground Substance

Collagen fibers in an extracellular matrix surround the cells. Collagen originates from the pulpal fibroblasts and is seen throughout the pulp. Both types I and II collagen have been found in the pulp. Type I is probably produced by the odontoblast, since dentin, which this cell forms, also consists of type I. Type II is probably produced by the pulp fibroblasts. In the young pulp, the fibers are relatively sparse and the tissue appears delicate (see Figure 9.12). Around the fibers is the ground substance of the pulp. This substance is the environment that promotes life of the cells in the pulp and throughout the body. If the pulp is irritated, fibers may accumulate rapidly. However, the older pulp contains more collagen of both the bundle and diffuse types (Figure 9.17).

Vascularity

The pulp organ is extensively vascular, with vessels arising from the external carotids to the superior or inferior alveolar arteries. It drains by the same veins. Although the periodontal and pulpal vessels both originate from these vessels, their walls are quite different. The walls of the periodontal and pulpal vessels become very thin as they enter the pulp. This is because the pulp is protected within a hard, unyielding container of dentin. These thin-walled arteries and arterioles enter the apical canal and pursue a direct route up the root pulp to the coronal area (Figure 9.18). Along the way, they give off branches that pass peripherally to a plexus that lies adjacent to the odontogenic zone of the root (Figure 9.19).

Blood flow is more rapid in the pulp than in most areas of the body, and the blood pressure is quite high. The diameter of the arteries varies from 50 to 100 μm, which equals the size of the arterioles in other areas of the body.

These vessels have three layers: the inner lining, or **intima,** which consists of oval or squamous-shaped endothelial cells surrounded by a closely associated fibrillar basal lamina; a middle layer, or **media,** which consists of muscle cells from one to three cell layers thick (Figure 9.20); and an outer layer, or **adventitia,** which comprises a sparse network of collagen fibers forming a loose network around the larger arteries.

Smaller arterioles with a single layer of muscle cells range from 20 to 30 μm, and **terminal arterioles** of 10 to 15 μm are also present. **Precapillaries** measuring 8 to 12 μm and **capillaries** 8 to 10 μm in diameter are present in the peripheral pulp. The capillaries are endothelium-lined tubes that form a network among the odontoblasts (see Figure 9.19). Numerous investigators have shown that lymphatic vessels are also present in the pulp. These vessels are thin-walled, irregularly shaped, and larger than capillaries and have an incomplete lamina supporting the intima and media.

■ Clinical Comment

The vitality of the pulp is due, in part, to the apical canal's ability to remain open. This opening can become blocked, however, as the tooth ages and cementum becomes deposited around the apical canal. Thin walls of veins are the first structure affected by cemental constriction of the apices; vascular congestion can occur, leading to pulpal necrosis.

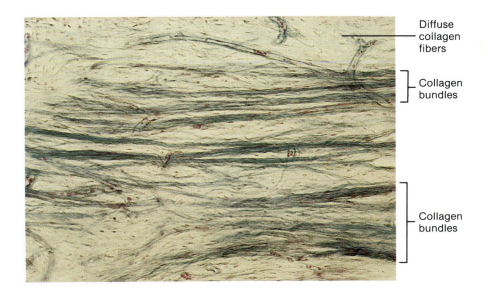

Diffuse collagen fibers

Collagen bundles

Collagen bundles

Figure 9.17 *Collagen bundles in an older pulp organ. Trauma was probably the cause of the bundles in this pulp.*

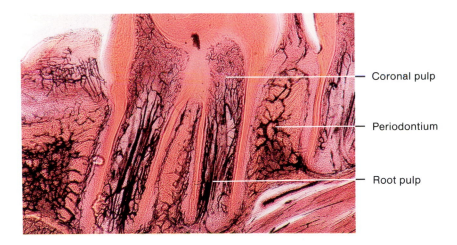

Figure 9.18 *Blood vascular organization in pulp and periodontium (India ink injection of vessels).*

- Coronal pulp
- Periodontium
- Root pulp

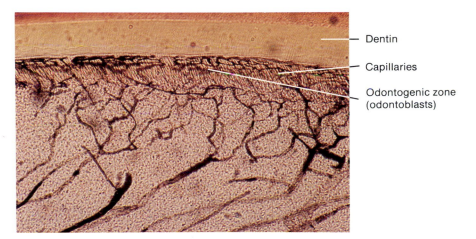

Figure 9.19 *India ink was injected into these blood vessels to illustrate the network of capillaries among the odontoblasts. Dentin is seen at the top of the picture and central pulp in the lower part.*

- Dentin
- Capillaries
- Odontogenic zone (odontoblasts)

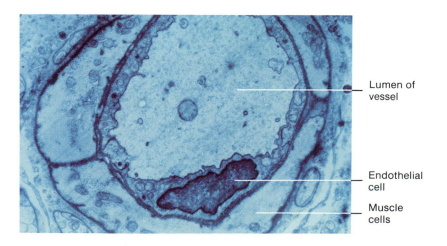

Figure 9.20 *Ultrastructure of pulp arteriole. Its central lumen is surrounded by endothelial cells; a nucleus is seen below. This is the intima layer. Surrounding the intima is a layer of muscle cells that comprises the media. External adventitial fibers are also present.*

- Lumen of vessel
- Endothelial cell
- Muscle cells

Nerves

Several large nerves enter the apical canal of each molar and premolar, and single ones enter the anterior teeth. These trunks traverse the radicular pulp, proceed to the coronal area, and branch as they extend peripherally (Figure 9.21). Nonmyelinated axons also enter with the myelinated axons, but they are smaller. A young premolar may have as many as 350 to 700 myelinated axons and 1,000 to 2,000 nonmyelinated axons entering the apex.

The large nerve trunks are all invested with Schwann cells (see Figures 9.14 and 9.15). Later, as the pulp organ matures, the subodontoblastic plexus is apparent only in the roof and lateral walls of the coronal pulp and, to a lesser extent, in the root canals. This network, composed of both myelinated and nonmyelinated axons, is known as the parietal layer of nerves or nerve plexus (Figures 9.21 and 9.22). From the parietal layer, the nerves pass into the odontogenic zone and then terminate among the odontoblasts and in the dentinal tubules.

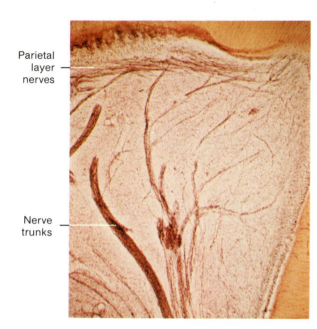

Parietal layer nerves

Nerve trunks

Figure 9.21 *Nerve trunks pass from the radicular pulp into the coronal zone. These nerves extend out to the periphery, where they form a plexus of nerves adjacent to the odontogenic zone at the top of the micrograph.*

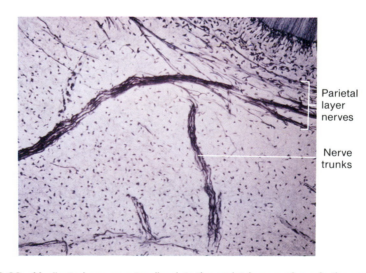

Parietal layer nerves

Nerve trunks

Figure 9.22 *Myelinated nerves extending into the parietal nerve plexus in the peripheral pulp. From this area they extend between the odontoblasts to terminate among them or in the predentinal tubules.*

Nerve Endings

Most of the pulpal nerve endings are in the odontogenic region of the pulp horns. Some terminate on or in association with the odontoblasts (Figures 9.23 and 9.24). Others are found in the predentin tubules of the crown (Figure 9.24). These endings are presumed to function in pain reception. Few nerve endings are found among the odontoblasts of the root. However, nerve endings are located along the larger muscular blood vessels in the central pulp. All these nerve endings have a similar appearance and are highly vesicular, but they are believed to function in constriction or dilation of large blood vessels of the pulp.

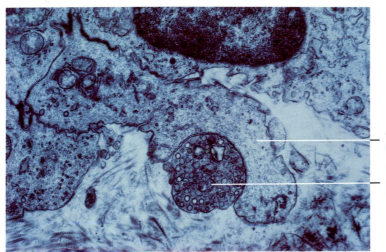

Odontoblastic process

Nerve ending containing vesicles

Figure 9.23 *Ultrastructure of a nerve ending in close contact with an odontoblastic process in the predentin. It contains small vesicles that probably contain neurotransmitter substance.*

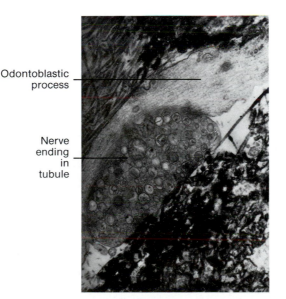

Odontoblastic process

Nerve ending in tubule

Figure 9.24 *Vesiculated nerve terminal in a dentinal tubule in contact with the odontoblastic process.*

■ *Pain and the Pulp-Dentin Complex*

Pain is a function of the high concentration of nerve endings within the tooth. Pulp is highly sensitive to temperature changes, electrical and chemical stimuli, and pressure as applied to the inner enamel, dentin, or pulp. Teeth are one of the few bodily structures that perceive only the modality of pain. The close relationship between the nerve endings and the odontoblasts and their processes is significant. Moreover, the nerve terminals in the tubules of the predentin and along the surface of the pulp are far from the area where pain is perceived, at the dentinoenamel junction and the inner enamel.

A second theory, called the **direct innervation theory,** was based on the belief that nerves extend to the dentinoenamel junction. However, no nerves were found at this junction when dentin was viewed with the electron microscope.

Some scientists, however, believe that the odontoblastic process is the receptor and in turn conducts the painful stimuli to these endings in the peripheral pulp or predentin. This has been termed the **transduction theory** (Figure 9.25).

A third theory, the **hydrodynamic theory,** was developed to explain the transmission of pain through the thickness of dentin (Figure 9.25). This theory is based on the premise that when the odontoblastic process is stimulated, it moves within the tubule contacting the nerve endings in the inner dentin and adjacent pulp. When these nerve endings are contacted, they deform and act as mechanoreceptors. Supporting this theory is the observation that the odontoblastic process and the nerve endings are closely related and interdigitating (see Figure 9.24). Substantial evidence has shown that when one stimulates the dentin with cold, the odontoblastic processes move outward, and when heat is applied, the odontoblast and its processes move inward. Dentinal fluid movement has been measured by the cutting of a tooth, an air blast, and application of a dry, absorbent paper.

The odontoblast is therefore a unique cell, forming dentin throughout its life and at the same time responding to various stimuli by acting on nerve endings in the tubules and peripheral pulp.

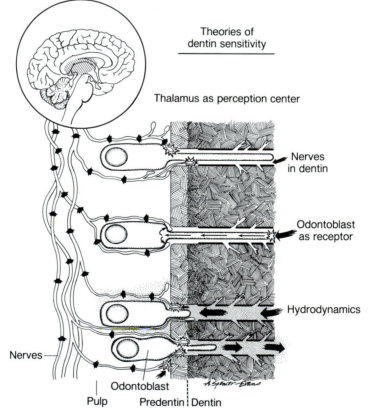

Theories of dentin sensitivity

Thalamus as perception center

Nerves in dentin

Odontoblast as receptor

Hydrodynamics

Nerves

Odontoblast

Pulp Predentin Dentin

Figure 9.25 *Summary of information on passage of nerve impulses through dentin. At the top, impulses are shown stimulating nerves directly; this is termed the direct stimulation concept. In the center, the odontoblast is depicted as the receptor passing impulses on to the brain (transduction theory). At the bottom is the concept of the odontoblast moving. This causes contact with the nerve ending, which in turn is a mechanoreceptor; this is termed the hydrodynamic theory. A hot stimulus causes the odontoblast to move pulpward, and a cold stimulus causes outward movement.*

■ *Functions of the Pulp*

Pulp has several functions, none more important than providing vitality to the teeth with its cells, blood vessels, and nerves. The loss of the pulp after a root canal does not mean the tooth will be lost; on the contrary, the tooth will function without pain. The tooth, however, has lost its protective mechanism that the pulp nerves provide.

The pulp has several other functions. It is **inductive** because very early in development the future pulp interacts and initiates tooth formation. The pulp organ is **formative,** since the odontoblastic cells of the pulp form the dentin that surrounds and protects (Figure 9.26). The pulp is **protective,** responding to stimuli such as heat, cold, pressure, and operative cutting procedures of the dentin. Finally, the pulp has the ability to be **reparative,** (Figure 9.26) through its response to surgical cutting or to caries, by the formation of tertiary or reparative dentin. Formation of sclerotic dentin, the process of obliterating the dentinal tubules, is protective to the pulp, which maintains the vitality of the tooth.

■ *Clinical Comment*

A cracked tooth may result from masticatory impact on a hard object on the margin of a restoration. As a result, salivary organisms can penetrate the crack, causing inflammation, pain, and eventually pulpal pathosis.

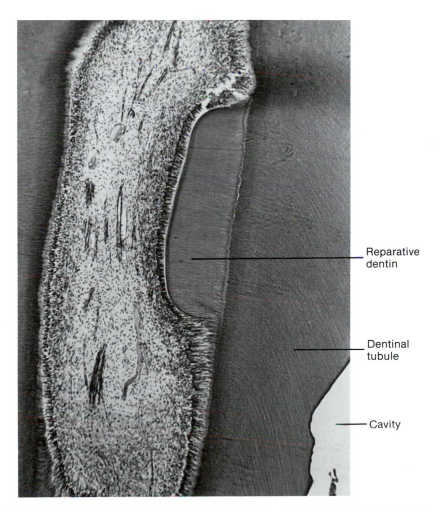

Reparative dentin

Dentinal tubule

Cavity

Figure 9.26 *Reparative dentin is deposited in the pulp underlying areas of stimulation by stimuli such as caries, abrasion, cavity preparation, and restorations.*

■ *Regressive Changes*

Numerous regressive changes in the pulp and surrounding dentin are related to environmental stimuli and to aging. It is often difficult to determine which factor has caused the specific change that is seen. As the tooth ages, the pulp decreases in size because of the continued deposition of dentin. This shrinkage generally occurs around the entire perimeter of the dentin (Figure 9.27). On the other hand, with attrition, abrasion, or operative procedures, there is appropriate deposition of dentin underlying the injured area (Figure 9.26). In addition, with both aging and injury, there are sclerotic changes or tubule occlusion within the dentin. In aging, deposition is generalized. Also with aging, the number of pulpal cells, the size of the perinuclear cytoplasm, and the number of organelles such as mitochondria and endoplasmic reticulum in these cells all decrease, indicating that cell activity has slowed. Therefore, aging decreases the ability of the pulp to respond to injury and to repair itself. With injury, however, deposition of dentin appears in a specific location (Figure 9.26).

Fibrous Changes

Fibrosis, which is seen in some pulps, is believed due more to injury than aging. In some cases, there is a diffuse fibrosis with collagen fibers throughout the pulp. Occasionally, the fibers nearly obliterate the pulp. What mechanism causes this process is not certain, although it is believed due, at least in part, to pulpal injury. Scarring caused by injury is an important factor. One characteristic of aging is an increase in collagen fibers, and with the decreasing size of the pulp these fibers become more evident (see Fig. 9.17). The reason why some pulps contain diffuse areas of collagen and others bundles of it probably relates to injury as well as to unknown systemic factors.

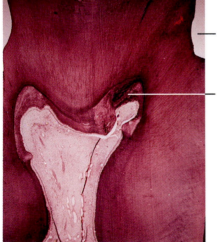

Cavity preparation

Reparative dentin

Figure 9.27 *Reparative dentin underlying a cavity preparation. Note the dentinal tubules of the floor of the cavity lead to the area where the reparative dentin is formed.*

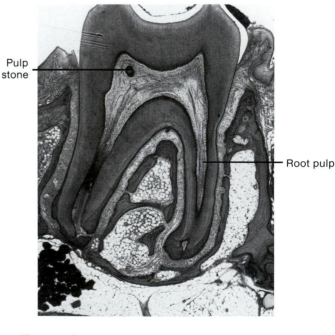

Pulp stone

Root pulp

Figure 9.28 *A free pulp stone appearing in the coronal pulp of a molar tooth.*

Pulpal Stones

Pulpal stones, or **denticles,** are round to oval calcified masses appearing in either the canal or coronal portions of the pulp organ (Figure 9.28). They appear in teeth that have suffered injury as well as in otherwise normal-appearing pulps. Pulpal stones also occur in unerupted as well as erupted teeth. These denticles are noted in most pulps of permanent teeth, especially in individuals more than 60 years of age. They are classified according to their structure as true or false. **True denticles** have dentinal tubules like dentin—hence the name *true.* Odontoblasts may be on the surface of the denticles, and their processes are evident in their tubules. **False denticles** are concentric layers of calcified tissue (Figure 9.29). In the center of these false stones may be a group of cells that appear necrotic. These cells are believed to serve as the nidus of denticle formation.

All denticles begin small and grow, sometimes nearly obliterating the pulp. Denticles may appear free in the pulp, attached to dentin, or embedded within dentin. Therefore, they are classified as **free, attached,** or **embedded denticles.** One pulp may have all three types (Figure 9.29). Investigators believe that a free denticle may become attached and, later, embedded as dentin is deposited around the denticle. The predominance of denticles are false ones and appear free in the pulp.

Diffuse Calcifications

Diffuse calcifications appear as irregular calcified deposits along collagen fiber bundles or blood vessels in the pulp. This is considered a pathologic condition and usually appears as a sprinkling or, occasionally, large masses of mineral. They appear more often in the root canal than the coronal area of the pulp.

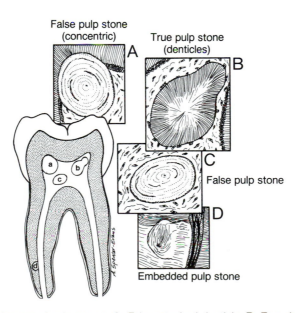

Figure 9.29 *Diagram of pulp stones.* **A.** *False attached denticle.* **B.** *True denticle with tubules.* **C.** *False, free denticle.* **D.** *Embedded denticle.*

■ Self-Evaluation Questions

1. What are the two most prominent cells in the pulp?
2. Name five other cell types found in the pulp.
3. Describe the characteristics of the odontogenic zone.
4. What specializations do the pulpal blood vessels exhibit?
5. What specializations do pulpal nerve endings exhibit?
6. Describe the nerve endings found in the pulp.
7. Name five functions of the pulp.
8. What are denticles?
9. Describe the two major types of denticles.
10. Where are these two types of denticles found?

■ Acknowledgments

Figures 9.1, 9.2, 9.5, 9.10, 9.13, 9.14, 9.21, 9.23, and 9.25 are from Chapter 5, Pulp, in Bhaskar, S.N., ed., *Orban's Oral Histology and Embryology,* St. Louis, C.V., Mosby, 1980.

Figures 9.9, 9.11, 9.12, 9.15, 9.19, 9.20, 9.22, 9.26, and 9.27 are kindly provided by Drs. D.J. Chiego, Jr., C.F. Cox, D.C. Johnsen, and D. F. Turner. These figures are reprinted from Avery, J.K., *Oral Development and Histology.* Toronto, B.C. Decker, 1988.

■ Suggested Reading

Avery, J.K. Oral development and histology. Toronto: B.C. Decker, 1988.

Avery, J.K. In: Bahaskar, S.N., ed. Orban's oral histology and embryology. St. Louis: C.V. Mosby, 1980.

Baume, L.J. The biology of pulp and dentine. In: Myers, H., ed. Monographs in oral science, vol. 8. New York: S. Karger, 1980.

Ten Cate, A.R. Oral histology, development, structure and function. St. Louis: C.V. Mosby, 1989.

Yamada, T., Nakamura, K., Iwaku, M., and Fusayama, T. The extent of the odontoblast process in normal and carious human dentin. J. Dent. Res. 1983; 62:798.

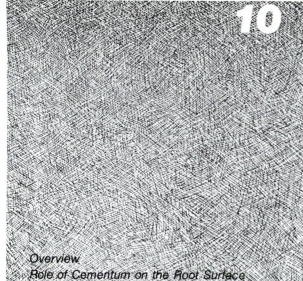

10

Cementum

■ Overview

Cementum, which is the focus of this chapter, has two major functions: sealing the tubules of the root dentin and serving as an attachment for periodontal fibers. Cementum has the ability to reverse resorption by means of deposition to form a smooth patch on the cemental surface.

Roots of the teeth are covered by two layers of very different types of tissue. The first, called intermediate cementum, is a homogeneous layer originating from root sheath cells. The second, called cellular cementum, is a thicker deposit of a cellular bonelike substance. The epithelial root sheath contributes to the intermediate cementum, and the cementoblasts differentiating from the periodontal ligament fibroblasts form cellular cementum. Cementum simulates bone by displaying cells within lacunae, canaliculi, cellular components, and incremental lines. Absent, however, are the vascular and the neural elements characteristic of bone. As a result, the cementum has unique characteristics, including lack of neural sensitivity and a greater ability than bone to resist resorption. Both of these are important clinical features. Aging cementum exhibits cementicles, which are similar to denticles in dentin in that they are calcified nodules that may be embedded, attached, or free.

■ *Role of Cementum on the Root Surface*

The hard tissue that covers the entire root surface is very thin, but it manages to carry out two important functions. First, it seals the surface of root dentin and covers the ends of the open dentinal tubules, and second, it attaches the periodontal fibers to the tooth. Sealing of the root surface is discussed in this chapter (Figure 10.1), while the attachment of fibers is presented in Chapter 12.

Two types of cementum are on the root surface. The first, called **intermediate cementum,** is a deposition by the epithelial root sheath cells formed during root formation before this cell layer disintegrates (Figure 10.2). The second is **cellular cementum,** the specialized hard tissue present on the root surfaces of teeth (Figure 10.2). Both grossly and histologically, cellular cementum resembles bone, since it is a hard, dense tissue with cells contained within lacunae and having canaliculi (Figure 10.3). How-

ever, unlike bone, cellular cementum does not contain blood vessels, nerves, **Haversian** or **Volkman's canals,** which are the nutrient canals containing the blood vessels and nerves in bone. Therefore, it is a characteristic of cellular cementum to be insensitive to pain. This cementum is more resistant to resorption than bone, and the lack of vascularity of cementum may be partially the reason. Although many blood vessels are near its surface, none actually enters. In laboratory tests, cementum is slightly more permeable to dyes than is bone or dentin. However, the permeability of live cementum is not known. Cementum is deposited in increments, so there are characteristic incremental lines similar to those of bone, dentin, and enamel (Figure 10.4). Although cementum has many characteristics of hard tissue, some elements are absent. Therefore, cementum is not exactly like any other tissue in the human body.

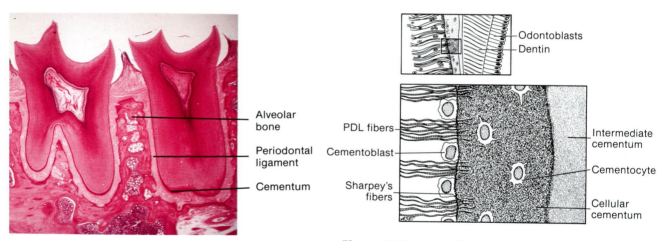

Figure 10.1 *Relation of the root to periodontium. Observe cementum on the root apex. The cementum covers the entire root surface overlying the granular dentin layers.*

Figure 10.2 *Intermediate cementum is on the right. Cellular cementum is seen in the center of the field and periodontal ligament (PDL) fibers on the left.*

Figure 10.3 *Early cementum deposition on root dentin. Observe that some cementoblasts get enmeshed in the cementum matrix and become cementocytes. They exist in lacunae.*

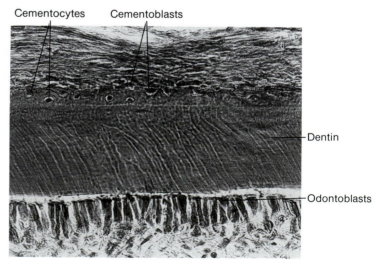

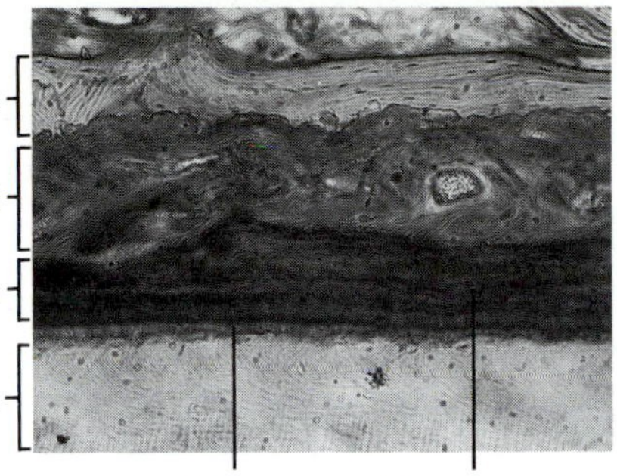

Alveolar bone

Periodontal ligament

Dental cementum

Dentin

Intermediate cementum Incremental line

Figure 10.4 *Histology of cementum on the root surface. Note the horizontal incremental lines in the cementum, which appear similar to bone, dentin, or enamel.*

Table 10.1   Relationship of Cementum to Enamel at Cementoenamel Junction

Relationship	Percentage of cases
Cementum overlaps enamel	60%
Cementum just meets enamel	30%
Small gap exists between cementum and enamel	10%

Cementum is limited to the roots of teeth. In 60 percent of cases, cementum is formed on the cervical enamel for a short distance; in 30 percent, it stops at the cervical line just meeting the enamel; and in 10 percent, there is a small gap between them. This order of frequency is known as the **OMG**—or overlap, meet, and gap. (Figure 10.5 and Table 10.1).

■ *Clinical Comment*

Cementum functions as a covering for the root surface, sealing the open dentinal tubules, and also as an attachment for the periodontal fibers that hold the tooth in its socket.

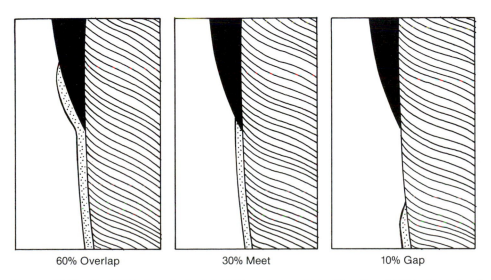

60% Overlap   30% Meet   10% Gap

Figure 10.5 *Relation of cementum to enamel at cementoenamel junction. OMG is the order of frequency of these conditions.*

■ *Intermediate Cementum*

Intermediate cementum is a thin, noncellular, amorphous layer of hard tissue 10 μm thick. It is deposited by the inner layer of the epithelial cells of the root sheath. Deposition occurs immediately before these epithelial cells disintegrate as a sheet and migrate away from the root into the periodontal tissues (Figure 10.6). Recently, several authors have used the term **intermediate cementum,** while others prefer **cementoid layer.** The latter term is confusing since the initial layer of cementum is called cementoid, like osteoid in bone. Intermediate cementum is the first layer of hard tissue deposited, and it seals the tubules of dentin. Because of its epithelial origin, intermediate cementum is composed of an enamelin protein rather than collagen, which is the protein typical of cellular or secondary cementum. Intermediate cementum is completely formed before deposition of the secondary cementum begins. As an amorphous, noncellular layer, it is similar to the aprismatic enamel layer on the crown surface of teeth. This cementum calcifies to a greater extent than either the adjacent cellular cementum or the dentin and therefore is of a harder consistency (see Figure 10.2).

■ *Cellular and Acellular Cementum*

Cementum is deposited directly on the surface of the intermediate cementum at a thickness of about 30 to 60 μm at the cervical region of the crown. It increases gradually to a thickness of 150 to 200 μm at the root apex (Figure 10.7). The cementum appears to be more cellular as its thickness increases, probably to maintain its vitality (Figure 10.8). The thin layer near the cervical region requires no cells to maintain vitality, because fluids bathe its surface.

Cementum forms more slowly than dentin, developing adjacent to it, as seen in Figure 10.6. After the inner epithelial root sheath cells stimulate the formation of the root dentin, and then deposit the primary intermediate cementum on the surface of this dentin, they quickly begin to degenerate and migrate from the root surface into the periodontal ligament. Then, the cementoblasts, which originate from the periodontal ligament, begin to form increments of cementum along the root surface.

Cementum is always thickest at the apex of the root (see Figure 10.7). As described in Chapter 5 on root development, cementum forms by depositing an increment of collagenous matrix that is secondarily mineralized. This matrix is called cementoid, and its formation is similar to that of bone from osteoid and dentin from predentin.

Some cementoblasts may become incorporated in the forming cementum along the developing front, as cementum continues to form around the cementoblasts (Figure 10.9; see Figure 10.2). These cells are then termed cementocytes because they reside in lacunae within the cementum. The greatest number of cementocytes in lacunae appear in the thick apical cementum (see Figure 10.8). The cementocytes found deep in the cementum are polygonal in appearance and have fewer organelles (Figure 10.10).

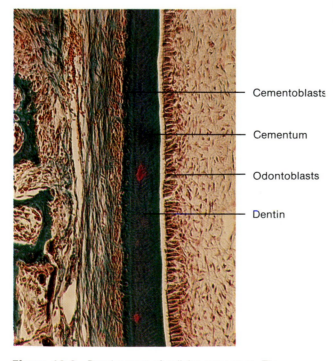

Cementoblasts

Cementum

Odontoblasts

Dentin

Figure 10.6 *Development of cellular cementum. The epithelial cells nest away from the root surface after forming the intermediate cementum.*

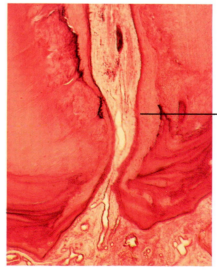

Cementum at root apices

Figure 10.7 *Thick cementum on root apices in an older person. Deposition of cementum around the apical canal may obliterate it, damaging the pulp.*

Deep within cementum, many lacunae appear empty, which implies that these cells gradually die. Some of these cells have long processes that lie in canaliculi and contact adjacent cementocytes (see Figure 10.9). Near the surface of cementum, the cells appear active with the organelles such as Golgi's apparatus, rough endoplasmic reticulum, and mitochondria, all associated with protein secretion (Figure 10.11). Layers of cellular and acellular cementum may alternate in their formation, although the reason is unknown.

The collagen fibers formed within the cementum are associated with the cementum's function on the root's surface. More superficially, cementum has bundles of noncalcified fibers that are associated with the function of attachment for the periodontal fibers. These fibers are spoken of as extrinsic fiber bundles of cementum.

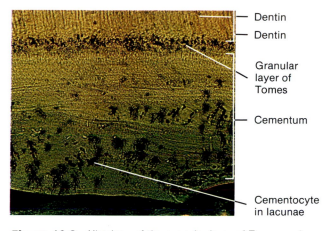

Figure 10.8 *Histology of the granular layer of Tomes and lacunae in the cementum. The greatest number of lacunae are found in the cementum near the apex.*

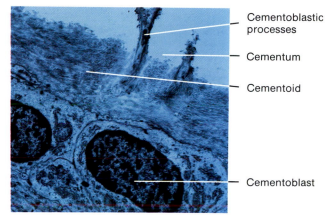

Figure 10.9 *Ultrastructure of early cementum. Cementoblasts become cementocytes as their processes become incorporated in the matrix. Cementocytes are located in cementum and do not appear in this photomicrograph.*

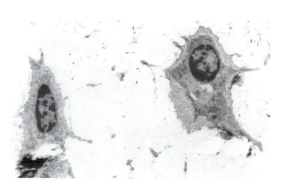

Figure 10.10 *Ultrastructure of two cementocytes deep in the cementum. These cells contain few organelles and appear to be inactive.*

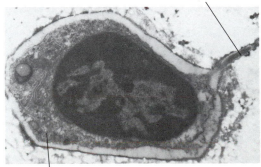

Figure 10.11 *Ultrastructure of a cementocyte near the surface of cementum. These cementocytes appear viable and relate to adjacent cementocytes by their processes.*

■ Physical Properties

As one group of hard connective tissues, cementum contains slightly less mineral than either bone or dentin (Table 10.2). It is slightly less hard than dentin. It is light yellow and can be distinguished from enamel, since cementum, unlike enamel, has no luster. However, cementum is slightly lighter in color than dentin, which makes it difficult to distinguish between the two.

The organic matrix of cementum is composed of collagen and chondroitin sulfate, and its mineral component is hydroxyapatite.

Table 10.2 Organic and Mineral Composition of Cementum, Dentin, and Enamel

Substance	Percentage organic material	Percentage mineral
Cementum	50–55% (collagen and H_2O	45–50% (Calcium and phosphorus
Dentin	30% (collagen)	65.5%
Enamel	30–35% (enamelin)	60–65%

■ Aging of Cementum

With aging, the relatively smooth surface of cementum becomes more irregular (Figure 10.12). This is due to calcification of some ligament fiber bundles where they were attached to the cementum. Such occurrences appear on most surfaces of cementum but, to a greater degree, near the apical zone. In aging, a continuing increase of cementum in the apical zone may obstruct the apical canal (see Figure 10.7). Microscopically, only the lacunae near the surface have viable-appearing cells, whereas those deeper lacunae all appear to be empty. Cementum resorption is one characteristic of aging cementum (Figure 10.12). Resorption may begin, and then cementum may deposit in the defect, creating reversal lines. Resorption sites may appear in dentin as well (Figure 10.13). This area may be covered with cementum later.

■ Clinical Comment

Cellular cementum appears similar to bone in structure, but does not contain any nerves. Therefore, cementum is nonsensitive. Scaling, when necessary, does not produce pain.

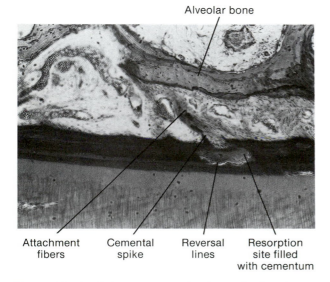

Figure 10.12 Aging cementum showing projection of spikes into the ligament. Note the reversal line (upper right). Cementum builds up around bundles of attachment fibers.

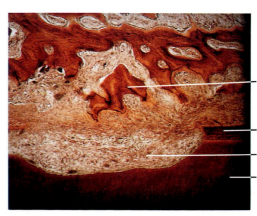

Figure 10.13 Cemental and dentin resorption with periodontal soft tissue occupying this area. Note that alveolar bone develops in this space compensating for root loss. The length of periodontal fibers is thus maintained.

Cementicles appear near the surface of aging cementum. Like denticles (discussed in Chapter 9) cementicles may be free, attached, or embedded (Figures 10.14 and 10.15). They are usually ovoid or round and exhibit concentric rings because of being formed incrementally. Cementicles are usually found in the periodontal ligament as it ages, either near the surface or embedded in the cementum, but in some cases they may be seen in a younger person after local trauma. Repair of cementum and dentin is a normal healing process. Attachment fibers then reappear (Figure 10.15).

■ Clinical Comments

Cementum is resistant to resorption. For this reason, tooth movement results in bone resorption, with minimal cemental loss. Cementum can also repair itself as well as areas of dentinal resorption. When resorption stops and cementum deposition begins, a *reversal line* can be seen (Figure 10.16). This line represents the reversal of the resorptive/formative process.

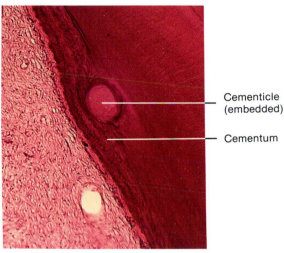

Cementicle (embedded)

Cementum

Figure 10.14 *Attached or embedded cementicles. Cementicles may be found free as small, round, calcified nodules in the ligament. They may also be embedded deep in the cementum.*

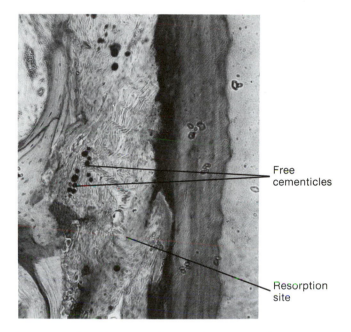

Free cementicles

Resorption site

Figure 10.15 *Free cementicles in the periodontal ligament. Observe the resorption area in the cementum on the right.*

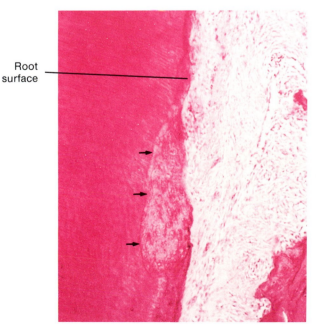

Root surface

Figure 10.16 *Reversal line in cementum is indicated by the arrows on the left. The root surface is again smooth as a result of this repair.*

■ Self-Evaluation Questions

1. What is the function of cementum?
2. What is the origin of intermediate cementum (cementoid)?
3. Where on the root is cementum thickest and thinnest?
4. Name three types of cementicles.
5. What does a cemental reversal line represent?
6. Is cementum less easily resorbed than bone, and what are the possible reasons?
7. In what percentages does cementum overlap with, meet, or gap from enamel?
8. Does cementum have nerves or blood vessels, and if so, what is the clinical significance?
9. What is the origin of cementoblasts and cementocytes?
10. Name two characteristics of aging cementum.

■ Acknowledgments

Figure 10.2, 10.6 and 10.9 are provided by Drs. N.M. Elnesr and J.K. Avery from Chapter 8 in Avery J.K., ed., *Oral Development and Histology,* Toronto, B.C. Decker, 1988.

Figures 10.1, 10.3, 10.5, 10.7, 10.8 and 10.10 through 10.16 are provided by J.K. Avery from Chapter 21, Histology of the Periodontium, in *Oral Development and Histology.*

■ Suggested Reading

Elnesr, N.M., and Avery, J.K. Development and root and supporting structures. In: Avery, J.K., ed. Oral development and histology. Toronto: B.C. Decker, 1988.

Lindskog, S. Morphology and formation of intermediate cementum in monkey (thesis). Stockholm: Karolinska Institute, 1982.

Scott, J.H., and Symons, N.B. Introduction to dental anatomy, 7th ed. Edinburgh: Churchill Livingstone, 1974.

Ten Cate, A.R. Development of the periodontium. In: Ten Cate, A.R., ed. Oral histology development, structure, and function. St. Louis: C.V. Mosby, 1989.

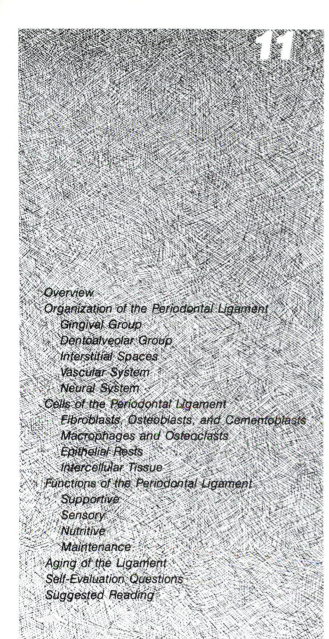

Periodontium: Periodontal Ligament

■ Overview

The periodontal ligament is a fibrous connective tissue ligament located between the alveolar bone proper and cementum. This ligament covers the root of the tooth and connects with the tissue of the gingiva. The periodontal ligament occupies the periodontal space and is composed of cells and intercellular substance. The latter consists of collagen fibers and ground substance, which in turn contains protein and polysaccharides. The periodontium develops from the dental follicle tissue that surrounds the tooth. In turn, the follicle gives rise to the cells forming the ligament fibers, the alveolar bone, and the cementum. It has a thickness of 0.15 to 0.38 mm, is thinnest in the midroot zone, and decreases slightly in thickness with aging. It is composed of collagen fiber bundles that attach the cementum to the alveolar bone proper. Interstitial spaces contain the blood vessels and nerve trunks that communicate freely with vessels and nerves of the alveolar bone. This tissue is highly cellular, containing fibroblasts and vascular, neural, bone, and cemental cells. The primary function of the periodontal ligament is support for the teeth, transmitting neural input to the masticatory apparatus, and its nutritive function is essential to maintaining the ligament's health, which has important clinical implications.

■ *Organization of the Periodontal Ligament*

Groups of principal fibers are named according to their location with respect to the teeth. There are two groups: the **gingival group,** located around the necks of teeth, and the **dentoalveolar group,** which surrounds the roots of teeth (Figure 11.1). These principal fibers are bundles of collagen fibers strategically positioned at inclinations important to their function along the root surface, from the cervical region to the tooth's apex, numbers 1 to 6 (Figure 11.1). The collagen fiber bundles are embedded in the cementum of the tooth root and extend into the alveolar bone. Therefore, they act as a suspensory ligament for the teeth.

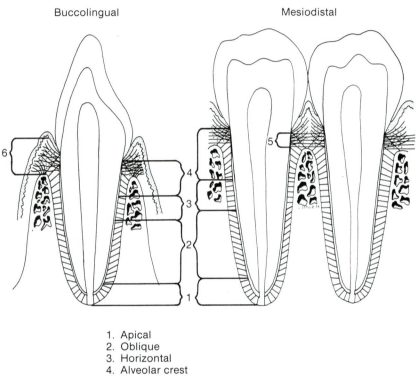

Buccolingual   Mesiodistal

1. Apical
2. Oblique
3. Horizontal
4. Alveolar crest
5. Transseptal
6. Gingival group

Figure 11.1 *The principal fiber groups of the periodontal ligament. All of the fibers listed in the buccolingual plane are also present in the mesiodistal plane. The transseptal fiber group, however, is seen only in the mesiodistal plane.*

Between each group of fibers is a space termed the **interstitial space** (Figure 11.2*A* and *B*). These spaces contain a network of blood vessels, nerves, and lymphatics that maintain the vitality of the periodontal ligament. Also, a network of finer fibers interlace and support the dense collagen bundles. They may be important since the collagen fibers are being stretched and contracted constantly during mastication.

The majority of supportive fibers are collagenous, but a few have been described as elastic-like and of a structure different from collagen. These are termed **oxytalan fibers** (Figure 11.3). Oxytalan fibers are small in diameter and appear to interlace with the collagen bundles, supporting the collagen fibers and the blood vessel walls as well. These very fine elastic-like fibers stain with special stains, which reveal their location to be almost longitudinal in the ligament when viewed through a light microscope (Figure 11.3).

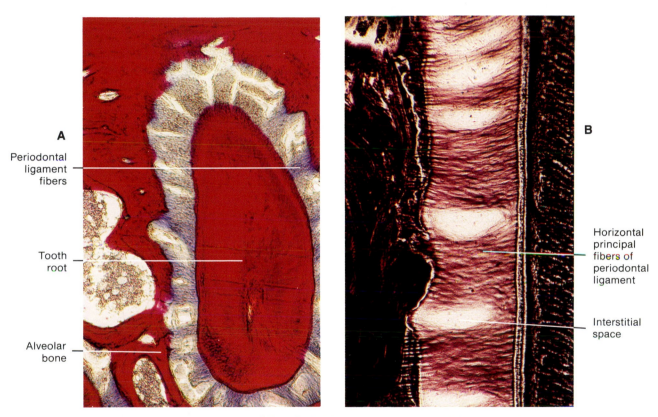

A

Periodontal ligament fibers

Tooth root

Alveolar bone

B

Horizontal principal fibers of periodontal ligament

Interstitial space

Figure 11.2 (A) *Appearance of the principal fiber bundles and interstitial spaces in the periodontal ligament in cross section.* (B) *The periodontal ligament and interstitial spaces in the plane longitudinal to the tooth.*

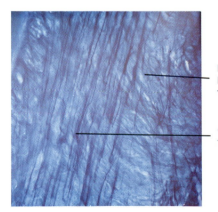

Periodontal ligament fibers

Oxytalan fibers

Figure 11.3 *Histologic appearance of longitudinally oriented oxytalan fibers in the periodontal ligament.*

Gingival Group

The fiber bundles of the gingival group represent four groups of principal fibers, each having a different orientation and function in support of the gingival tissues (Figure 11.4). The **free gingival** fibers arise from the surface of the cementum in the cervical region and pass into the free gingiva to provide support. The **attached gingival** fibers also arise from the alveolar crest and pass into free and attached gingiva; they provide support. The **circular** or **circumferential** fibers, continuous around the neck of the tooth, resist gingival displacement. The **aveolar crest** fibers arise from the cementum and proceed to the bone of the alveolar crest. The **transseptal fiber group** originates in the cervical area of each crown and extends to a similar area on the mesial or distal only on these surfaces of an adjacent tooth (Figures 11.5 and 11.6). This fiber group functions as resistance to the separation of teeth. It is noted in Figure 11.6 that transseptal fibers are found in the mesiodistal plane and are not present in the bucolingual plane. All of these fiber groups are illustrated in Figure 11.1 and listed in Table 11.1.

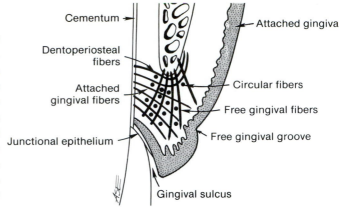

Figure 11.4 *The four groups of gingival fibers. The dentogingival fibers extend from the cervical cementum into the free and attached gingiva. The alveologingival fibers extend from the alveolar crest into the gingiva. The circular fibers surround the teeth, and the dentoperiosteal group extends from the cervical cementum into the alveolar crest.*

Table 11.1 Principal Fibers

Fiber group	Location of attachment	Function
Dentoalveolar Fiber Group		
Apical	Apex of root of fundic alveolar bone proper	Resist vertical forces
Oblique	Apical one third of root to adjacent alveolar bone proper	Resist vertical and intrusive force
Horizontal	Midroot to adjacent alveolar bone proper	Resist horizontal and tipping force
Alveolar crest	Cervical root to alveolar crest of alveolar bone proper	Resist vertical and intrusive force
Interradicular	Between roots to alveolar bone proper	Resist vertical and lateral movement
Gingival Fiber Group Transseptal	Cervical tooth to tooth mesial or distal to it	Resist tooth separation mesial distal
Attached gingival	Cervical tooth to attached gingiva	Resist gingival displacement
Free gingival	Cervical tooth to free gingiva	Resist gingival displacement
Circumferential	Continuous around neck of tooth	Resist gingival displacement

Dentoalveolar Group

The dentoalveolar group consists of five differently oriented types of principal fiber groups named according to their origin and insertion in the dentoalveolar process. The **alveolar crest group** originates at the cervical area just below the cementoenamel junction and extends to the alveolar crest as well as into the gingival connective tissue (Figure 11.6). These fibers resist intrusive forces. The **horizontal fiber group** extends in a horizontal direction, from the midroot cementum to the adjacent alveolar bone proper. These fibers resist tipping of the teeth, illustrated in Figure 11.7. The **oblique fiber group** extends in an oblique direction from the area just above the apical zone of

the root upward to the alveolar bone (Figure 11.8). These fibers resist vertical or intrusive masticatory forces. The **apical fiber group** extends perpendicular from the surface of the root apices to the adjacent **fundic alveolar bone,** which surrounds the apex of the tooth root. This group resists vertical and extrusive forces when applied to the tooth (Figure 11.8). The fifth group of fibers, located between the roots of the multirooted teeth, are called the **interradicular fiber group.** These fibers extend perpendicular to the tooth's surface and into the adjacent alveolar bone in multirooted teeth (Figure 11.9). They resist vertical and lateral movement. All of these fiber groups except the last are shown in Figure 11.1 and all are listed in Table 11.1.

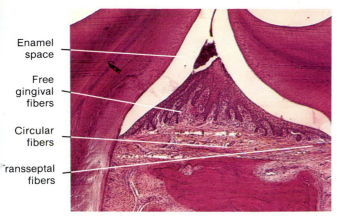

Enamel space

Free gingival fibers

Circular fibers

Transseptal fibers

Figure 11.5 *Histology of gingival fibers in the interproximal area. Observe the transseptal fiber group that extends from the mesial of one tooth to the distal of the adjacent tooth. Observe the relationship of the free gingival and the circular fibers to the transseptal fibers.*

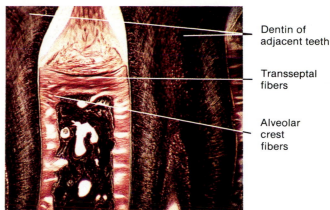

Dentin of adjacent teeth

Transseptal fibers

Alveolar crest fibers

Figure 11.6 *Histology of the alveolar crest fibers extending from the cementum of the cervical region to the alveolar bone. The periodontal fibers penetrate the alveolar bone. Also observe the transseptal fibers extending from the tooth on the left to the right.*

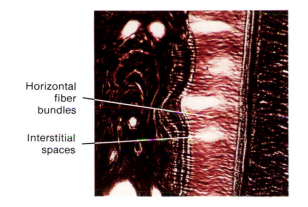

Horizontal fiber bundles

Interstitial spaces

Figure 11.7 *Histologic appearance of the horizontal fiber bundles. Observe that they are oriented perpendicular to the tooth surface and are embedded by perforating fibers in the cementum and alveolar bone.*

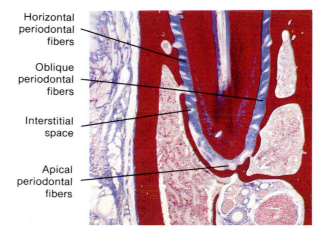

Horizontal periodontal fibers

Oblique periodontal fibers

Interstitial space

Apical periodontal fibers

Figure 11.8 *Histology of the horizontal, oblique, and apical fiber groups of the periodontal ligament. Observe the angulation of each series of bundles to resist forces of mastication.*

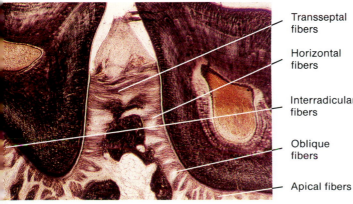

Transseptal fibers

Horizontal fibers

Interradicular fibers

Oblique fibers

Apical fibers

Figure 11.9 *Histology of the interradicular fiber groups located between the roots and alveolar bone of multirooted teeth.*

■ **Clinical Comment**

Health of periodontal tissue has major importance to the dental health of the patient and to dental functions. Today, interest in preventive periodontal care is expanding, as well as the use of various diagnostic skills.

Interstitial Spaces

The principal fibers make up the structural and functional bulk of the periodontal ligament. They are positioned at regular intervals along the gingival-apical extent of the periodontal ligament. Between each bundle of principal fibers an interstitial space appears. These spaces appear in both the cross-sectional and longitudinal planes of the ligament (see Figure 11.2). The regularity of these spaces clearly relates to the vascular and neural needs of the functioning ligament. Interstitial spaces appear designed to carry these vascular and neural structures both by encircling the tooth at intervals and by connecting with the vessels that run longitudinal to the root (see Figure 11.2B). These interstitial spaces are designed to withstand the impact of masticatory forces. The collagenous fiber bundles that surround these spaces are arranged at angles to the surfaces of the spaces, providing support for their maintenance. These spaces are compressed during mastication or tension as noted in Figure 11.10.

Vascular System

The periodontal ligament has a rich blood supply that arises from the inferior and superior alveolar arteries and branches of the facial artery from the external carotid. These vessels supply the alveolar bone and anastomose freely with the periodontal ligament. The vascular plexus that elongates into the ligament extends from the apical to the gingival areas with loops that surround the teeth at regular intervals (Figure 11.11A). The complexity of the vascular plexus is seen in Figure 11.11B, which illustrates the density of the ligament. When the alveolar bone and tooth have been sectioned and cleared and the vascular plexus injected with carbon particles, the relationship between these vessels of the alveolar bone and ligament is distinctly seen (Figure 11.12). Numerous arterioles and venules traverse the ligament in a well-organized network. There are numerous arteriovenous shunts in the ligament that provide direct connections between the arterial and venous blood supply without having to go through a capillary network. The ligament has been found to be an active site for cell turnover, tissue modification, and, in some cases, healing. These conditions relate to the rich vascular supply.

■ Clinical Comment

The suspensory apparatus of the teeth is organized to protect the blood vessels from compression. Pressure receptors in the ligament are protective to these tissues.

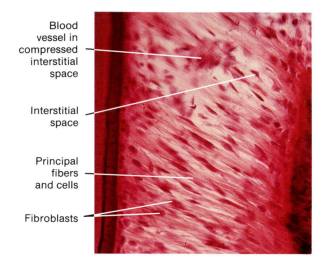

Blood vessel in compressed interstitial space

Interstitial space

Principal fibers and cells

Fibroblasts

Figure 11.10   *Histology illustrating the fibers, cells, and interstitial spaces in the periodontal ligament under tension.*

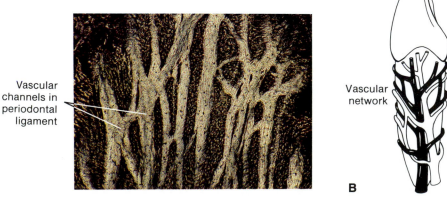

Vascular channels in periodontal ligament

Vascular network

A

B

Figure 11.11   (A) *Histology of the periodontal ligament illustrating the continuity of the network of the interstitial spaces that run longitudinally in the ligament with lateral connections throughout the ligament.* (B) *Diagram of the network of blood vessels in the ligament. Both arteries and veins vascularize the very active periodontal ligament.*

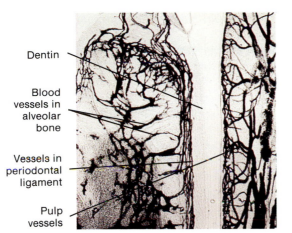

Dentin

Blood vessels in alveolar bone

Vessels in periodontal ligament

Pulp vessels

Figure 11.12 *Cleared alveolar bone and ligament after injection of vessels with carbon. Note the vessels from the bone on the left entering the ligament in the center of the field. Vessels in the tooth pulp can be seen on the right of the field.*

Neural System

The larger nerve trunks traverse the periodontal ligament in the central zone of the tooth's long axis (Figure 11.13). Branches pass into and from the alveolar bone into the ligament. Some nerves pass to the interstitial spaces, as seen in Figure 11.14. Pressure receptors are located among principal fibers of the ligament (Figure 11.15). These specialized neural endings are enclosed in a connective tissue capsule and function during masticatory movements of the jaw.

■ *Clinical Comment*

Maintaining normal tissue vitality through disease prevention and constant maintenance is imperative. Oral health is dependent on both continuous professional care and patient participation.

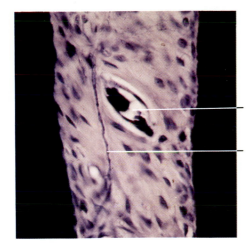

Interstitial space

Nerve trunk

Figure 11.13 *Nerve trunks perfusing the periodontal ligament to accompany blood vessels, function as receptors to pressure and pain, and provide vasoconstriction and dilatation.*

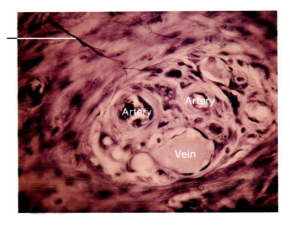

Nerve

Artery

Artery

Vein

Figure 11.14 *A high-magnification view of an interstitial space. Observe the nerve entering the interstitial space from the ligament (upper left). In the central oval area are arteries veins, and nerves.*

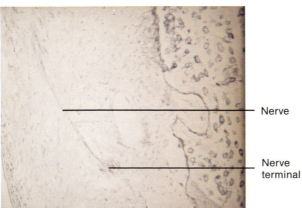

Nerve

Nerve terminal

Figure 11.15 *A nerve trunk attached to an oval nerve ending in the ligament. The nerve terminal appears to be a pressure receptor (modified pacinian). They have an important function in sensing the density of food during mastication.*

■ Cells of the Periodontal Ligament

Fibroblasts, Osteoblasts, and Cementoblasts

Several types of cells located in the ligament have formative, supportive, and resorptive functions. Fibroblasts are the most numerous cells seen in the periodontal ligament because of the high collagen density of this tissue. The abundance of fibroblasts allows rapid replacement of fibers (see Figure 11.10). Osteoblasts are located along the surface of the alveolar bone, and cementoblasts appear near the cementum. These cells differentiate locally from mesenchymal cells as the need for these cells arises.

Macrophages and Osteoclasts

Macrophages in the ligament, are important defense cells because of their phagocytic activity and mobility. They take up bacteria, dead cells, and foreign bodies.

Some fibroblasts form and destroy collagen. This process was described in Chapter 6 on tooth eruption. Collagen may form at one end of the cell and be destroyed at the other end (Figure 11.16). The fibroblasts have the ability to simultaneously synthesize and degrade collagen, a process essential to the periodontal ligament's high turnover of collagen. Fibroblasts maintain a balance of collagen formation and destruction in the ligament. Macrophages, lymphocytes, leukocytes, and plasma cells may also appear in the periodontium when it is stressed by disease.

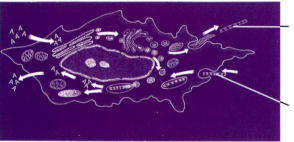

Formation of new fibers

Ingestion of collagen fibers and breakdown into amino acids

Figure 11.16 *Fibroblasts are present in the ligament in great numbers. It is probable that some of these cells function in forming as well as destroying collagen fibers as the need arises.*

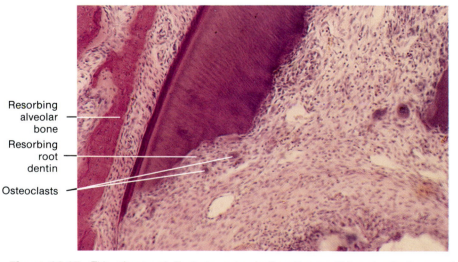

Resorbing alveolar bone

Resorbing root dentin

Osteoclasts

Figure 11.17 *This micrograph illustrates osteoclastic action modifying alveolar bone and root surface.*

Osteoclasts, in instances of tooth movement or periodontal disease, may function in bone resorption (Figure 11.17). They appear as a normal consequence of tipping or bodily movement of a tooth (Figure 11.18). Osteoclasts originate from monocytes within the blood vascular system and become the multinucleated cells seen in the lacunae of resorption sites in hard tissue (Figure 11.17).

Epithelial Rests

Epithelial rests are normal constituents of the periodontal ligament that are seen throughout life. Epithelial cells are scattered throughout the ligament, but in the early life of the tooth they are seen along its root surface. Epithelial rests may appear as resting, proliferating, or dividing cells, which means they go through periods of activity as well as periods when they may remain for unknown lengths of time before dividing. Their function is unknown. Epithelial rests are most evident when they are located along the root surface, as seen in Figure 11.19.

Intercellular Tissue

Intercellular tissue surrounds and protects the cells of the periodontal ligament and is also the product of these cells. This extracellular matrix (ECM) is composed of water, glycoproteins, and proteoglycans that surround the collagen fibers. These protein and polysaccharide substances provide the cells with vital substances that arise from the blood capillaries and return catabolites from these cells to the vessels.

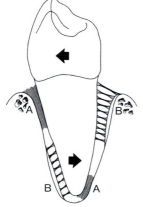

Figure 11.18 *Diagram of a tooth tipping which may occur in orthodontic tooth movement. As the tooth crown moves to the left, the root moves to the right. As ligament zone A is compressed, zone B is stretched.*

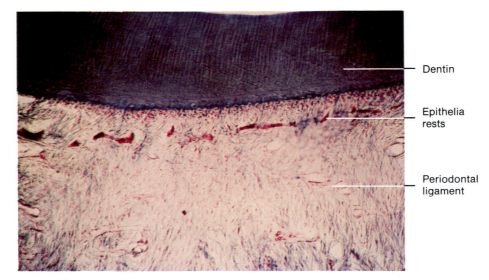

Dentin

Epithelia rests

Periodontal ligament

Figure 11.19 *Epithelial rests appear in the periodontal ligament near the cementum covering the dentin at the top of the micrograph.*

■ Functions of the Periodontal Ligament

Supportive

Possibly the most important function of the periodontal ligament is support of the teeth. Failure of this function results in tooth loss. Every time the teeth are clenched, as in mastication, the periodontal fibers are stretched and then relaxed. This system is highly efficient to compensate for the thousands of times this ligament is called into action.

Sensory

The periodontal ligament is supplied with abundant receptors and nerves that sense any movement in function. When the receptors sense pressure, the nerves send signals to the brain to inform the masticatory apparatus, including the temporomandibular joint and muscles of mastication.

Nutritive

The blood vessels of the ligament provide the essential nutrients for the ligament's vitality and the hard tissue of cementum and alveolar bone. All cells such as fibroblasts, osteoblasts, cementoblasts, and even the resorptive osteoclasts and macrophage cells require nutrition, which is carried by the blood vessels to the ligament (Figure 11.20).

When an orthodontic appliance causes compression and constriction of these vessels, soft tissue changes are first noted at the site, followed by loss of alveolar bone, which is necessary to allow space for blood flow to occur. The periodontium therefore responds as a coordinated unit.

Maintenance

Tissues are forming and responding rapidly in the masticatory apparatus. Interaction of cells with their intercellular environment is continuous. These tissues function for a lifetime, if health is maintained and appropriate care provided.

■ Clinical Comment

Renewal capability is an important characteristic of the periodontal ligament fibers. It provides for maintenance of the system and repair if needed.

■ Aging of the Ligament

Aging occurs in this tissue as in all other tissues of the body. There is a gradual decrease in cell number and cell activity as aging takes place. In aging cementum and alveolar bone, scalloping occurs (Figure 11.21). Fibers are attached to the peaks of these scallops rather than over the entire surface. This is one of the more remarkable changes that occurs in the aging of supportive structures of the teeth. Activity of these tissues is likely to decrease during the aging process because of restricted diets, and therefore, normal functional stimulation of these tissues is diminished. With aging, a healthier periodontium can result from general good health of the individual and good oral hygiene. A loss of gingival height related to gingival and periodontal disease promotes destructive changes. Unfortunately, at that time, the presence of a low-grade inflammation may be characteristic of the gingival tissue.

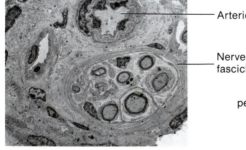

Figure 11.20 *Ultrastructure of interstitial space with nerve bundle* (lower right) *and arterioles* (above).

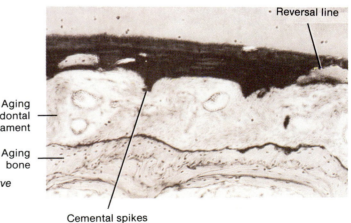

Figure 11.21 *Aging periodontal ligament, cementum, and alveolar bone. The fiber bundles of the ligament are decreased in number. Cemental and bone spikes are caused by excessive deposition around the few fiber bundles.*

■ Self-Evaluation Questions

1. Describe the principal fibers in the gingival fiber group of the periodontium.
2. Describe the five principal fiber types in the dento-alveolar group.
3. Define interstitial spaces.
4. Define the vascular system of the periodontal ligament.
5. Describe the nerves of the periodontal ligament.
6. What types of cells are found in the periodontal ligament?
7. What are epithelial rests, and where are they found?
8. What are the functions of the periodontal ligament?
9. Describe the characteristics of aging in the periodontal ligament.
10. Define oxytalan fibers.

■ Suggested Reading

Bernick, S., Levy, B., Dreize, S., and Grant, D.A. The intraosseous orientation of the alveolar component of marmoset alveodental fibers. J. Dent. Res. 1977; 56:1409.

Fullmer, H.M., and Lillie, R.D. The oxytalan fiber: A previously undescribed connective tissue fiber. J. Histochem. Cytochem. 1958; 6:426.

Fullmer, H.M., Sheetz, J.H., and Narkates, A.J. Oxytalan connective tissue fibers: A review. J. Oral Pathol. 1974; 3:291.

Melcher, A.H. Periodontal ligament. In: Bahaskar, S.N., ed. Orban's oral histology and embryology. St. Louis: C.V. Mosby, 1986.

Simmons, T.A., and Avery, J.K. Electron dense staining affinities of mouse oxytalan and elastic fibers. J. Oral. Pathol. 1980; 9:183.

Ten Cate, A.R., and Deporter, D.A. The role of the fibroblast in collagen turnover in the functioning periodontal ligament of the mouse. Arch. Oral Biol. 1974; 19:339.

Periodontium: Alveolar Process and Cementum

12

■ Overview

The periodontium is composed of four supporting tissues: gingiva, bony alveolar process, cementum, and periodontal ligament. This chapter describes the relationship of the bony and cemental supports to the periodontal ligament. The alveolar process is the bony part of the maxilla and mandible that has the primary function of supporting the teeth. Alveolar bone is compared to alveolar bone proper and supporting bone. The alveolar bone proper is the attachment for the periodontal ligament fibers. The continual turnover of alveolar bone and cementum results in resorption and deposition and maintains these structures as well as changes related to tooth movement. Tipping, rotation, and bodily movement of teeth performed by the orthodontist result in resorption of alveolar bone proper and cementum along the advancing root surface and deposition along the opposite surface of the root. Both cementum and bone closely coordinate their activities in this matter. These two hard tissues change with increased or decreased function and with aging. An old cemental or alveolar bone surface is denser and has fewer fiber bundles than a young one. As calcification occurs around some of these bundles, a scalloped surface of the hard tissue is created on the bone or cemental surface. Loss of bone from the alveolar process results in tooth loss, which in turn results in edentulous jaws.

■ *Alveolar Process*

The alveolar process is that part of the maxilla and mandible that supports the roots of teeth and is composed of **alveolar bone proper** and **supporting bone** (Figure 12.1). The alveolar bone proper is the bone lining the tooth socket. In clinical radiographic terms, it is called the **lamina dura.** This is the site of attachment for the periodontal ligament fibers. Supporting bone is the remainder of the alveolar process, specifically the compact cortical plate on the outer surface of the alveolar process, the spongy bone between the cortical plates, and the alveolar bone proper (Figure 12.2) The alveolar process develops as a result of tooth development and root elongation. Alveolar bone matures as the teeth gain functional occlusion, and it continues to function throughout life and disappears only when the teeth are lost. The teeth are responsible for not only the development but also the maintenance of the alveolar proc-

ess of the mandible and maxilla. The coronal border of the alveolar process is known as the **alveolar crest** (Figure 12.2). It is located about 1 to 1.5 mm below the cementoenamel junction of the teeth. This crest is rounded in the anterior region and nearly flat in the molar area. If the teeth are in buccal or lingual position, the alveolar process may be thin or missing. The area of bone loss where an apical root penetrates the bone is known as a **fenestration,** and bone loss in the coronal root zone is termed **dehiscence** (Figure 12.3).

■ *Clinical Comment*

The lamina dura is an important diagnostic landmark in determining the health of the periapical tissues. Loss of density usually means infection, inflammation, and resorption of this bony socket lining.

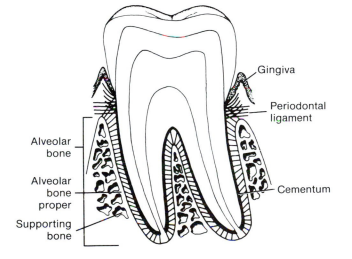

Figure 12.1 *The alveolar bone proper, supporting bone, and cementum of the periodontium.*

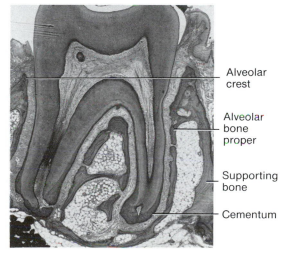

Figure 12.2 *Histology of the tooth and its supportive tissues. Note the relationships among the alveolar bone proper, the supporting bone, and the cementum covering the roots.*

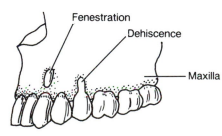

Figure 12.3 *Loss of alveolar bone adjacent to the tooth. Loss near the root apices is termed fenestration, and bone loss in the region of the coronal root is termed dehiscence.*

Alveolar Bone Proper

The compact or dense bone that lines the tooth socket is of two types when viewed microscopically. This bone either contains perforating fibers or appears similar to compact bone found elsewhere in the body. The perforating fibers, or **Sharpey's fibers,** are bundles of collagen fibers embedded in the surface of the alveolar bone proper at right angles or oblique to its surface along the entire long axis of the tooth (Figure 12.4). The fiber bundles inserting in the bone are regularly spaced and appear similar to those that insert into the root surface cementum (Figure 12.5). These perforating fibers are not unusual to periodontal bone and appear elsewhere in the body, where ligaments or tendons attach to cartilage or bone.

Since bone of the alveolar process is regularly penetrated by collagen bundles, it has been appropriately given the name **bundle bone.** Therefore, bundle bone is synonymous with alveolar bone proper, or **lamina dura,** and appears more dense radiographically than the adjacent supportive bone (Figure 12.6). This density is probably due to the mineral content or orientation of the bone crystals around the fiber bundles. Blood vessels and nerves penetrate the lamina dura through small foramina, but the mineral density is sufficient so that this bone appears opaque in radiographs (Figure 12.6). Tension on the perforating fibers during mastication is believed to stimulate this bone. This is thought to be important in its maintenance.

Not all alveolar bone proper appears as bundle bone, however, because this bone lining the socket is constantly being modified for adaptation to the stresses of occlusal impact. New bone is formed that does not have perforating fibers (Figure 12.7). Also, teeth are continually moving (drifting) within their sockets. Fibers may be lost or gained in various areas of the root and bone as a result of this action.

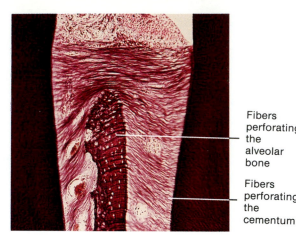

Fibers perforating the alveolar bone

Fibers perforating the cementum

Figure 12.5 *Histology of perforating (Sharpey's) fibers. Note the uniformity of position of the numerous fibers on the cemental and bony surfaces. The fiber bundles of the bone are larger and less numerous than those in the cementum.*

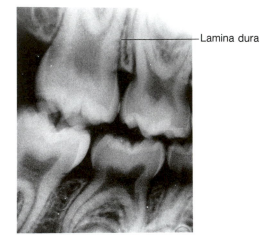

Lamina dura

Figure 12.6 *Radiograph of the alveolar bone illustrating the lamina dura, that radiodense bone lining the tooth sockets.*

Foramen between periodontal ligament and bone marrow

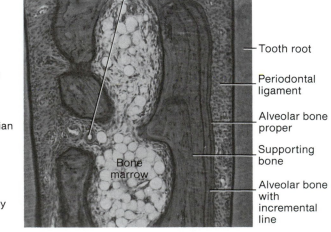

Tooth root

Periodontal ligament

Alveolar bone proper

Supporting bone

Bone marrow

Alveolar bone with incremental line

Figure 12.7 *Histology of alveolar bone proper and supporting bone. Note the foramina communicating between the periodontal ligament and the marrow space in the supporting bone on the left.*

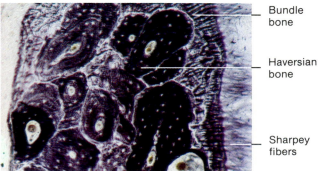

Bundle bone

Haversian bone

Sharpey fibers

Figure 12.4 *Histology of the alveolar crest area illustrating bundle bone with penetrating (Sharpey's) fibers and Haversian-type supporting bone.*

Supporting Compact Bone

Supporting compact bone of the alveolar process is similar to **Haversian bone** found elsewhere in the body (Figure 12.8). This compact bone of the alveolar process extends over the buccal or labial surface and the lingual surface of the mandible or maxilla (see Figures 12.1 and 12.2). Compact or cortical bone contains osteons with radiating lamellae accentuated with lacunae, which are connected with characteristic canaliculi (Figure 12.9). The haversian and **Volkmann's canals** form a continuous system containing the blood vessels that communicate between the hard and soft tissues. Bone cells, or osteocytes, may be present in many of the lacunae of compact bone, and they communicate with other osteocytes by means of small tubelike channels termed **canaliculi** (see Figure 12.9).

Supporting Cancellous Bone

The cancellous or spongy bone supporting the alveolar bone proper of the alveolar process is composed generally of heavy trabeculae, or plates of bone with bone marrow spaces between. Bone marrow contains blood-forming elements, osteogenic cells, and adipose tissue (see Figure 12.7). The supporting bone of the maxillae in particular is filled with marrow tissue, which contains immature red blood cells and leukocytes, especially in the molar region posterior to the maxillary sinus. Bone marrow, found in bones throughout the body, is the largest organ in the body, representing approximately 4.5 percent of body weight.

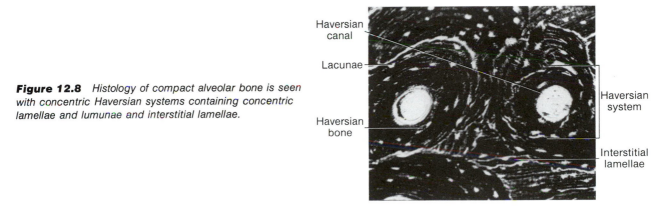

Figure 12.8 *Histology of compact alveolar bone is seen with concentric Haversian systems containing concentric lamellae and lumunae and interstitial lamellae.*

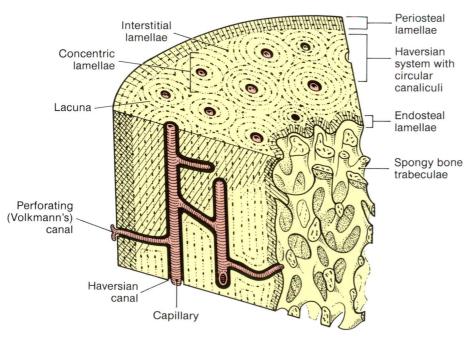

Figure 12.9 *Haversian system of compact bone similar to compact bone throughout the body. Observe the periosteal lamellae that would cover the surface of the mandible and the numerous haversian systems containing blood vessels and nerves interconnected by Volkmann's canals. The lacunae containing osteocytes surround the haversian canals.*

■ Cemental Support

Cementum functions in support by means of the attachment to perforating fibers of the periodontal ligament. The surface to the cementum has the appearance of bundle bone because of the perforating fibers over the entire surface of the roots (see Figure 12.5). Some areas of the cementum are inactive, with an absence of fiber bundles, or they undergo surface resorption (Figure 12.10). The collagen fiber bundles of cementum are more numerous than the bundles arising from the alveolar bone proper (see Figure 12.5). A similar level of attachment, however, is believed to be established on both the tooth and bone surfaces.

One characteristic of the surface of cementum is its ability to resorb; however, this occurs less often and to a smaller degree than it does in the alveolar bone proper. This characteristic of comparatively less resorption and repair is of clinical importance since it allows tooth movement without loss of the roots' protective covering. Some investigators claim an autoinvasive factor in cementum contributes to its resistance. Others believe the resistance is due to the absence of a blood supply in cementum as there is in bone. The distribution of the penetrating fibers over the surface of cementum could relate to this as well. Cementum will resorb, however, as does dentin during exfoliation of the primary teeth. Root loss is considered a normal process, described as a physiologic root and cementum loss due to permanent tooth eruption. Surface resorption may also occur as a result of tooth drift or traumatic occlusion, as described subsequently in this chapter.

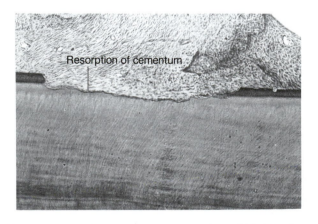

Resorption of cementum

Figure 12.10 *Cemental loss by resorption, which has also destroyed the adjacent bone.*

■ Tooth Movement

Physiologic

The eruptive process involves major remodeling of the alveolar process to compensate for root growth and changes in positional relations of the primary and permanent teeth. Repositioning of teeth occurs, for example, during facial growth. Movement occurs in facial and buccal directions as the arches increase in dimension (Figure 12.11). The height of the alveolus increases in relation to root growth as part of the facial growth process. There is an accommodation for increased dimension of the permanent teeth. In one situation, space is created in the arches by the replacement of larger primary molars by smaller permanent premolars. This is known as **leeway space** (Figure 12.12). This important situation helps compensate for the **incisor liability** factor, which is the replacement of the small primary incisors with larger permanent ones (Figure 12.13A and B). Part of this increase is compensated for by the inclination of the permanent incisors (Figure 12.13B). Also important is the **mesial drift,** a significant occurrence during this mixed dentition period. When the teeth are clenched during normal masticatory function, an anterior force is exerted on the teeth because most cusps are inclined anteriorly and their occlusal inclined planes therefore produce an anterior force. This is due in part to approximal wear. Summation of these forces defines the principle of mesial drift of the teeth.

The alveolar process compensates for tooth-related factors such as increased arch size in growth as well as effects of occlusal function. The effect of tooth loss or hypereruption is mesial drift, which would result in disruption of normal occlusal function.

■ Clinical Comment

The rate of mesial drift varies from 0.05 mm to 0.7 mm per year. This may relate to dietary factors and age.

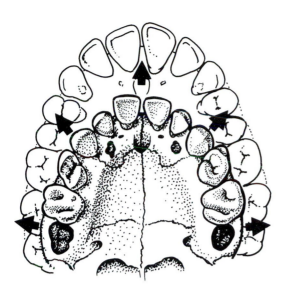

Figure 12.11 *Growth of the face results in migration of the teeth laterally and anteriorly and the increasing dimension of the arch posteriorly as the permanent molars develop and erupt.*

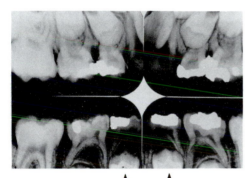

Permanent premolars

Figure 12.12 *A radiograph and histologic section of a permanent premolar replacing a primary molar. The smaller premolar produces a leeway space in the arch.*

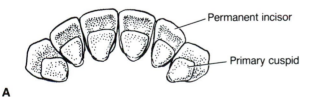

Permanent incisor

Primary cuspid

A

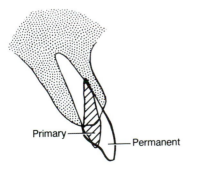

Primary — Permanent

B

Figure 12.13 *(A) Comparison of the interdental spacing of primary and permanent teeth. (B) Comparison of inclination of anterior primary and permanent teeth.*

Orthodontic

Tooth movement by orthodontics is possible only if bone resorption takes place in the direction in which the tooth is being moved. Such movement causes pressure on that surface of the alveolar bone in the direction of tooth movement. Tooth movement also causes tension on the periodontal ligament on the opposite surface of the root. These stresses cause activation of cells and changes in the vascular and neural tissue along the bone and cemental surfaces, which are mediated through the periodontal ligament (Figure 12.14). The alveolar bone and cementum show remarkable ability to be modified. As bone resorption occurs on one surface of the lamina dura or bone lining the tooth socket, the tooth is allowed to move in that direction, and bone concurrently forms on the opposite side of the socket. This stabilizes the tooth in the new position.

For example, if a tooth is tipped, as seen in Figure 12.15A, several areas of the periodontium are compressed and several exhibit tension. The **tipping** movement is necessary to accomplish the change in occlusion desired. Pressure applied at a specific point on the tooth causes compression in a limited area between the root and bone. However, a tooth may need to be moved by **bodily movement,** in which case the root is moved in the same direction, affecting the entire surface of the socket. Compression changes occur in the ligament along the advancing root surface, and tension changes occur in the ligament fibers, bone, and cementum along the opposite surface (Figure 12.15B). The situation is the same whether a single-rooted tooth or a multiple-rooted tooth is involved. In the multiple-rooted tooth, movement is complicated by the bifurcation bone, which has the additional bony surface related to pressure and tension (see Figure 12.14).

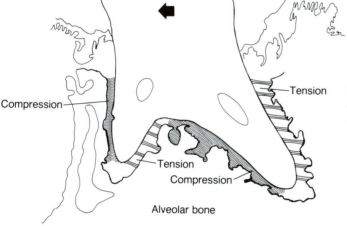

Figure 12.14 *Tooth movement to the left, with zones of compression along the advancing root surface and tension along the trailing root surface.*

Figure 12.15 (A) *Tipping of a tooth crown to the left causes the root to compress (C) the ligament at upper left and lower right. Tension (T) occurs at upper right and lower left. (B) Bodily movement of the crown and root to the left causes compression of the ligament, bone resorption along the entire surface of the advancing root, and bone formation of the tension surface on the right.*

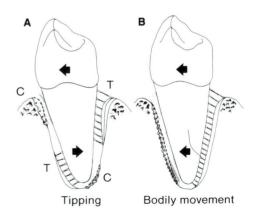

When compression is too great or too rapid, it causes **hyalinization** of the ligament. The vascularity is excluded, and the ligament appears colorless or "hyalinized." Tooth movement is limited by the rate of resorption, meaning cells that respond to the needs of compression and tension must be mobilized. On the compression surface, bone removal is the requisite, so osteoclasts must become organized. These cells originate from monocytes in the blood stream. The osteoclasts mobilize rapidly, appearing within a few hours after tooth movement begins (Figure 12.16).

Bone loss may occur on the bony surface of the socket, on the cementum of the root surface, or on both. This action may be reversed by deposition of bone or cementum in the area of resorption. The process of deposition in a resorption zone is known as an **area of reversal.**

On the tension side of the root, collagen fibers appear stretched, and the cells become oriented in the direction of the tension (Figure 12.17). The number of fibroblasts and osteoblasts increases (Figure 12.17). As this occurs, the force of tension is transmitted into a biologic force characterized by the appearance of cells that are responsive to these needs. Fibroblasts, osteoblasts, and cementoblasts arise from mesenchymal cells in this area and begin to function. Many fibroblasts are present to function in collagen renewal. Osteoblasts in turn synthesize bone proteins necessary for osteoid, and they also mineralize the bone matrix. As tension continues, bone is produced along the alveolar bone and cemental surfaces around the stretched perforating fibers (Figure 12.18).

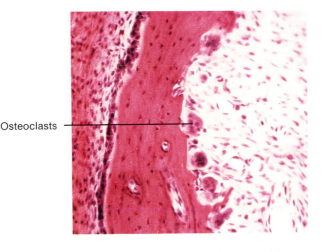

Osteoclasts

Figure 12.16 *Histology of the compression zone of the periodontal ligament. Observe that the osteoclasts remove bone to relieve the compression.*

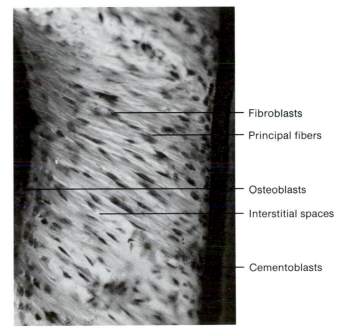

— Fibroblasts

— Principal fibers

— Osteoblasts

— Interstitial spaces

— Cementoblasts

Figure 12.17 *Histology of the tension zone of the periodontal ligament. Observe the stretched fibers and the number of osteoblasts and cementoblasts along the surface of the hard tissue.*

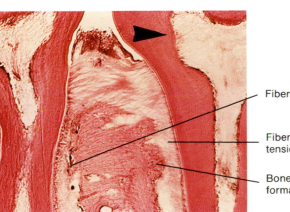

Fibers in compression

Fibers in tension

Bone formation

Figure 12.18 *Interproximal zone of two molar teeth. Tooth movement to the right (arrowhead) causes compression of the ligament on the left and tension on the right. Bone formation appears along the alveolar bone on the right as a result.*

Other types of tooth movement include rotation and a combination of tipping and rotation. In addition, intrusion or extrusion of a tooth may be needed. Figure 12.19*A* and *B* illustrates a case of tooth movement over a long term. Note the finger-like projections of bone following the path of tooth movement. This was the result of tension. The principles of compression and tension are similar in all cases. The plasticity of the alveolar process is remarkable.

■ *Clinical Comment*

Patients may be concerned about tooth mobility even when it is within normal limits. Teeth are slightly more mobile in the morning than later in the day.

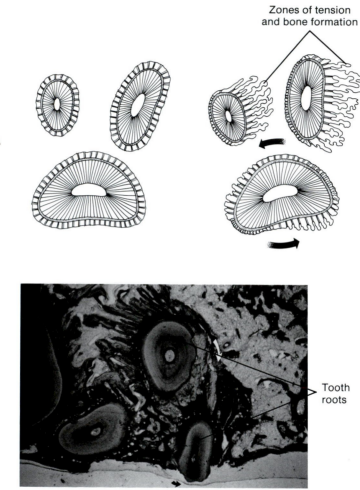

Figure 12.19 (A) *Rotation of a maxillary molar. The large lower root moved less than the upper two roots. Observe the bone formed along the trailing root surfaces and resorption on the advancing bony surface.* (B) *Histology of rotation of a maxillary molar illustrating loss of bone along the advancing surfaces and bone formation along the tension (trailing) surfaces. In addition to rotation, the tooth is moving away from the zones of tension?*

■ Aging of Alveolar Bone and Cementum

A comparison of young and old alveolar bone reveals a shift with age from dense bone and smooth-walled sockets to osteoporotic bone and sockets with rough, jagged walls. With aging, there is bone loss with fewer fiber bundles being inserted in the bone and cementum. Hard tissue then forms around the fibers in support of these bundles, which creates a scalloped surface (Figure 12.20). During aging there are fewer viable cells in the lacunae, and the marrow spaces become infiltrated with fat cells. Osteoporosis then becomes more apparent, and support of the teeth is further diminished.

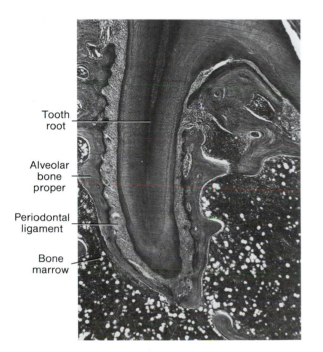

Tooth root

Alveolar bone proper

Periodontal ligament

Bone marrow

Figure 12.20 *Histology of aging alveolar bone illustrating scalloping of the alveolar bone proper.*

■ Edentulous Jaws

Several facts are known about the loss of teeth, although much remains to be learned about the changes in the bony alveolar process after tooth loss. First, it is recognized there is a decrease in alveolar bone volume. This is evident from the general loss of the alveolar process with tooth extraction. Next, there is some loss of the internal structure of the bone, resulting in open spaces and fewer trabeculae in the cancellous supporting bone (Figure 12.21). Osteoporosis may then become more evident. Little change occurs in the location of blood vessels, nerves, glands, and fatty zone in the aging edentulous jaws.

■ Clinical Comment

Physiologic tooth movement can be monitored through radiographic examination, and changes in the interproximal bone density or dimension can also be evaluated. The orthodontist relies on radiographs obtained in various planes to follow bone resorption and formation. Radiographs are also useful in following bone changes in the aging patient. Recognizing changes in the gingival and alveolar mucosa is another valuable index of tissue health.

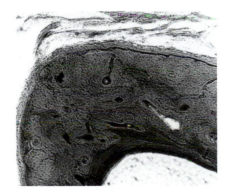

Figure 12.21 *Histology of edentulous jaws with loss of the tooth-bearing alveolar bone. The compact bone of the mandible is dense, and there is little evidence of osteoporosis at this stage.*

■ Self-Evaluation Questions

1. Describe the life length of alveolar bone.
2. What type of bone forms most of the lamina dura?
3. Cortical plates are classified as what type of alveolar bone?
4. What is the origin of osteoclasts and osteoblasts?
5. Describe the tension aspect of tooth movement and the type of cells that are activated.
6. Describe the compression aspect of tooth movement and the type of cells that are activated.
7. Define mesial drift.
8. Describe changes expected in the aging periodontium.
9. Define an area of reversal in cementum or alveolar bone.
10. Define tipping and bodily movement with regard to tooth movement.

■ Acknowledgment

Figure 12.13 provided by Dr. D.C. Johnson. In Oral Development and Histology, Toronto, B.C. Decker, 1988.

■ Suggested Reading

Berkovitz, B.K.B., Moxham, B.J., and Newman, H.N., eds. The periodontal ligament in health and disease. Oxford, UK: Pergamon Press, 1982.

Furseth, R. The fine structure of the cellular cementum of young human teeth. Arch. Oral Biol. 1969; 14:1147.

Jones, S.J., and Boyde, A. A study of human root cementum surfaces as prepared for an examination in the scanning electron microscope. Z. Zellforsch. 1972; 130:318.

Lisodeskog, S., and Hammerstrom, L. Evidence in human teeth of anti-invasive factor in cementum or perio ligament. Scand. J. Dent. Res. 1980; 88:161.

Mark, B.I. The microanatomy of the human edentulous maxillae. Aust. Dent. J. 1978; 23:69.

Melcher, A.H., and Bowen, W.H., eds. The biology of the periodontium. New York: Academic Press, 1969.

Severson, J.S., Moffett, B.C., Kokich, V., and Selipsky, H. A histologic study of age changes in the adult human periodontal joint (ligament). J. Periodontol. 1978; 49:189.

13 Temporomandibular Joint

■ Overview

The temporomandibular joint (TMJ), an articulation between the condyles of the mandible and the temporomandibular fossa of the temporal bone, is covered in this chapter. This joint allows the mandibular condyles to move in both gliding and hinge actions. Therefore, instead of being a stationary hinge, the joint moves along an inclined plane while functioning as a hinge joint. The complex motion of this joint has been observed during mastication. TMJ problems have been signaled by pain in the associated muscles of the head and neck.

The anatomy, histology, and function of the various structures composing this joint are reviewed in this chapter. The TMJ has several parts: (1) two condylar heads on the right and left sides of the mandible, (2) the articulating surfaces of the temporal fossa, (3) a disc that intervenes between the condyle and the fossa, and (4) a capsule and supportive ligaments. The capsule enclosing this joint serves as a stabilizer, making complex function possible. An articulating disc divides the joint into two halves—an upper, involved in a sliding action, and a lower, which functions in a hinge action. The joint is supported anteriorly by a tendinous attachment of the capsule and the lateral pterygoid muscle, laterally by the lateral or temporomandibular ligament, medially to a lesser extent by the sphenomandibular ligament, and posteriorly by the stylomandibular ligament. The TMJ functions as a ginglymoarthrodial joint, indicating that it moves as a sliding and hinge joint.

Myofacial pain dysfunction (MPD) syndrome has been defined as a complex problem that has received attention relating to neuromuscular concepts, occlusal concepts, muscle balance, tooth morphology, condylar guidance, and psychophysiologic factors. Much remains to be learned about the normal and abnormal stomatognathic system.

■ *Structure*

Condyles

Both the right and left heads of the condyles articulate in the glenoid or temporomandibular fossa. In adults they are ovoid in shape, and consist of a smooth bony surface covered with fibrous connective tissue (Figure 13.1). From birth to maturity, the heads of the condyles are generally round, gradually gaining the ovoid shape as they approach age 25 years. The condyles grow laterally during development.

From birth to adulthood, the condyles are covered with cartilage, which gradually thins. Initially, this cartilage serves as a growth site of the condyle as new cartilage cells differentiate from the perichondrium. Cartilage cells grow and divide near the surface of the condyle, and then the cartilage cells deeper in the condyle die and the surrounding cartilage calcifies (Figure 13.2A). Gradually, the cartilage layer is replaced by bone from below (Figure 13.2B). This process continues until only a thin cartilage layer remains, and at maturity the cartilage is replaced by bone (Figure 13.2C).

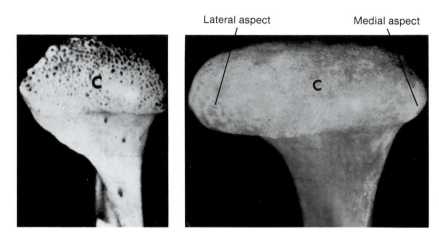

Figure 13.1   (Left) *A 6-year-old condyle (C). Observe the perforations on the surface created by the cartilage, which is missing because of tissue preparation.* (Right) *An adult bony smooth-surface condyle (C). Note the lateral growth.*

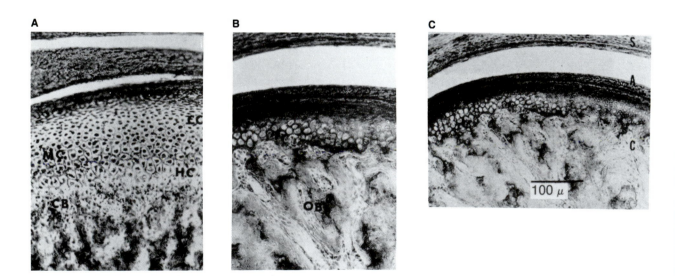

Figure 13.2   (A) *Histology of the condyle showing a wide band of cartilage appearing in the postnatal period. EC = reserve cartilage zone; MC = multiplication cartilage zone; HC = hypertrophy cartilage zone; and CB = calcifying zone.* (B) *The cartilage has thinned considerably. OB = bone formation.* (C) *A thin cartilage zone underlying the perichondrium at age 18 years.*

The head of the condyle and the head of long bones differ in that the long bones do not form secondary ossification sites (Figure 13.3). Secondary ossification sites produce epiphyseal lines where the lengthening of long bones occurs. However, the head of the condyle does accomplish growth like a long bone by the differentiation of new chondroblasts, the growth of the cartilage matrix, and replacement by bone. In long bone, the cartilage cells are in long rows scattered in the condyle. This cartilage-bone junction is a site of growth in height for the mandibular condyles (Figures 13.2 and 13.3). The anterosuperior slope of the bilateral condyles serves as the articulation with the eminence of the TMJ temporal bone. The heads of the condyles undergo morphologic adaptation to functional stress.

Temporomandibular Fossa

The fossa is composed of an anterior part, in the form of an eminence, and a posterior part, a depression or cavity on the inferior aspect of the temporal bone. This fossa is located at the posterior medial end of the zygomatic arch (Figure 13.4). In the anterior area are located the articular eminences—smooth, rounded ridges or tubercles, on whose posterior slope the condyles slide during articulation. On the posterior wall of the fossa is the petrotympanic fissure, from which elastic fibers are attached that insert into the posterior part of the disc. These elastic fibers may function in retroactive action of the disc. Anterior to this fissure is the articular fossa, that area of the temporomandibular fossa in which the condyles are positioned at rest (Figure 13.4).

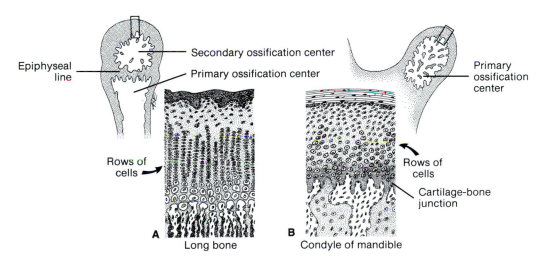

Figure 13.3 (A) *Cartilage of long bone.* (B) *The condyle. In A, note the straight rows of cartilage cells, young to maturing ones, top to bottom. In B, note the random cell arrangement, accomplishing the same function.*

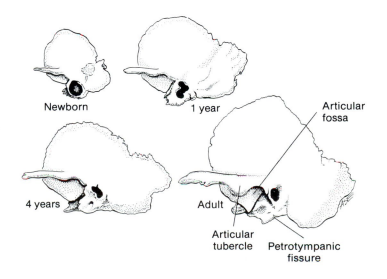

Figure 13.4 *Development of the glenoid (temporomandibular) fossa from birth to maturity.*

Upper and Lower Compartments

The temporomandibular joint cavity is divided into upper and lower compartments by the articular disc (Figure 13.5). The upper compartment is bound by the articular fossa and below by the disc. The lateral, medial, anterior, and posterior boundaries form the capsule that encloses the TMJ. The lower compartment is bound superiorly by the disc and below by the head of the condyle. The two compartments differ in action. In the upper compartment, there is a gliding action between the condyle head and the articular eminence, and in the lower compartment, there is a hinge action between the undersurface of the disc and the rotating surface of the condyle head (Figure 13.5).

Articular Disc

The articular disc is a dense, collagenous, fibrous pad between the condylar heads and the articular surfaces (Figures 13.5 and 13.6). When the jaw opens, the head of each condyle rises from the two articular fossae and slides anteriorly on the articular eminence along the intervening articular disc (Figure 13.7A). The head of the condyle rotates during the sliding motion, as seen in Figure 13.7B. This allows for the two movements of smooth **gliding** action and **hinge** action of the TMJ. The disc is thin and avascular in its center and thicker around the margins (Figure 13.8). The articular disc attaches to the inner wall of the capsule anteriorly and posteriorly but not medially and laterally, where it attaches to the head of the condyle. This structural design determines why the disc rotates when the head of the condyle moves.

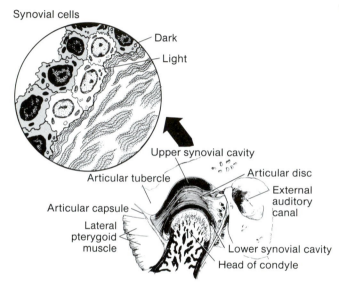

Synovial cells

Dark

Light

Upper synovial cavity

Articular tubercle

Articular disc

Articular capsule

External auditory canal

Lateral pterygoid muscle

Lower synovial cavity

Head of condyle

Figure 13.5 *Histology of the temporomandibular joint with the thick and thin parts of the articular disc, the location of the capsule anteriorly and posteriorly, the compartments and the relation to the lateral pterygoid muscle, and the external auditory canal. The upper and lower compartments are both lined with synovial cells. There are two types of cells: light and dark. They function to lubricate the movements of the condyles in the fossae.*

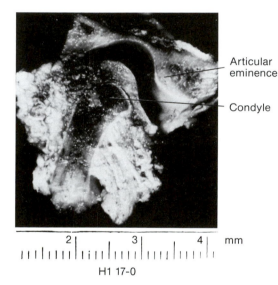

Articular eminence

Condyle

2   3   4   mm

H1 17-0

Figure 13.6 *Lateral view of the gross appearance of a temporomandibular joint at 17 years of age.*

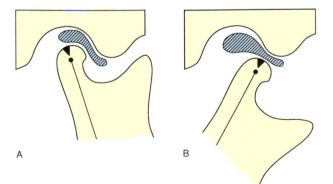

A   B

Figure 13.7 *The two actions of the temporomandibular joint. (A) The pathway of movement of the condylar head along the slope of the articular eminence. (B) The rotary movement of the condyle as the mouth is opened. Both actions occur simultaneously.*

The disc is covered with a thin layer of cells, or **synovial membrane,** that secretes a synovial fluid moistening the articular pad and surfaces of both upper and lower compartments (Figure 13.9). The synovial membrane is associated with numerous capillaries and lymphatics along the surface of the disc's perimeter. Synovial fluid is a distillate of the blood, having a high viscosity providing lubrication. The disc may perforate in its thin center or the center may contain a few cartilage cells and/or islands of cartilage, especially in older age.

■ *Clinical Comment*

The TMJ is a complex and precisely integrated bilateral joint that functions in speech and deglutition. One can perceive the downward and forward sliding action of the condylar heads by placing the fingers on them and opening the jaw. This sliding action can also be felt during symmetrical protrusion and retrusion or asymmetrical lateral shift.

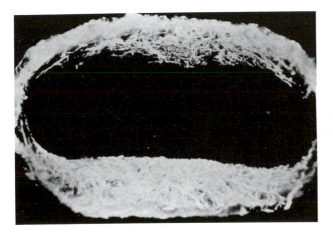

Figure 13.8 *The articular disc with the vascular channels injected with latex and the surrounding tissue removed. This method illustrates that the vascular network is only in the periphery of the disc and avascular in its center.*

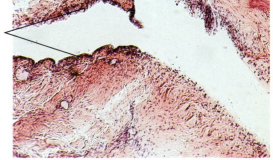

Synovial cells

Figure 13.9 *Histology of the soft tissue lining the TMJ cavities illustrating the synovial cells that line the joint.*

Capsule and Ligaments

A fibrous capsule encloses the TMJ like a cuff. This capsule is composed of an inner lining or synovial layer and an outer tough, but loose fibrous ligamentous tissue that supports the articulatory movements. The attachment superiorly is to the temporal bone around the limits of the articular eminence and the fossa, and it attaches around the neck of the condyle (Figure 13.10A). Fibers of the capsule fuse with the fibers of the lateral pterygoid muscle anteriorly, and laterally the capsule is strengthened by the lateral, or **temporomandibular,** ligament (Figure 13.10B). Medially, the **sphenomandibular ligament** supports the joint (Figure 13.10C). This ligament arises superiorly from the spine of the sphenoid bone and extends downward on the medial side of the ramus to insert on the lingula, which is a spine of bone arising from the rim of the mandibular foramen (Figure 13.10C). Posteriorly, the **stylomandibular ligament** arises from the styloid process and inserts on the posterior border of the ramus (Figure 13.10B and C). The lateral ligament and the capsule work in concert to support the joint and limit excursions of the condyles to the normal range. The other two ligaments, the sphenomandibular and stylomandibular, are supportive in nature. Mandibular movements are an interplay of the morphology of the teeth and the action of the muscles and ligaments.

Vascular Supply

The blood supply to the TMJ is from four sources: (1) branches of the **superficial temporal,** (2) **deep auricular,** (3) **anterior tympanic,** and (4) **ascending pharyngeal arteries** (Figure 13.11). All of these vessels converge on the joint, penetrate the capsule, and send branches into a network of vessels in the periphery of the disc and posterior area of the joint. Observe in Figure 13.11 that the disc is oval and has more blood vessels in the posterior and anterior areas than on the lateral surfaces. Interestingly, the blood vessels do not enter the fibrous covering of the heads of the condyle as do blood vessels in some other joints.

Innervation

The nerve supply to the TMJ arises from branches of the mandibular division of the trigeminal nerve—the **auriculotemporal, masseteric,** and **deep temporal** branches (Figure 13.12A to C). These are the same nerves supplying the muscles of mastication that function with this joint. Both large myelinated and smaller nonmyelinated nerves enter the capsule and disc, and they supply all four surfaces of the condyle heads, fossa, disc, and capsule (Figure 13.12). Pain, temperature, touch, and deep pressure terminals are located in the joint. Elaborate encapsulated terminals have been found in the connective tissue associated with the synovial folds and the disc. Four types of terminals located in the TMJ are shown in Figure 13.13.

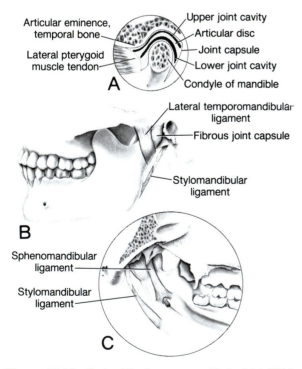

Figure 13.10 *Parts of the temporomandibular joint (TMJ). (A) The TMJ compartments and capsular ligament. (B) The lateral and posterior ligaments of the TMJ. (C) The medial ligament of the TMJ.*

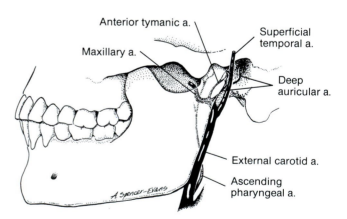

Figure 13.11 *Vascular supply to the temporomandibular joint. The joint is supplied by the external carotid, by branches of the ascending pharyngeal and the superficial temporal. The maxillary artery gives rise to the deep auricular and anterior tympanic arteries to the joint. (a = artery.)*

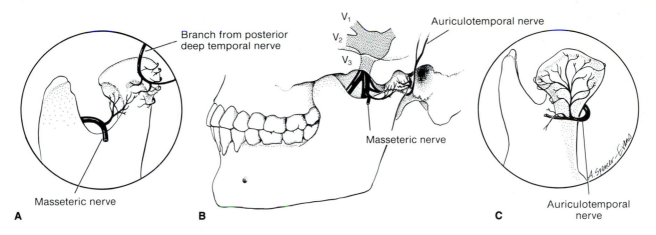

Figure 13.12 *Nerve supply to the temporomandibular joint. The mandibular division of the fifth nerve supplies all surfaces of the joint through the auricular temporal, masseteric, and deep temporal branches. (A) Anterior view; (B) lateral view; (C) posterior view.*

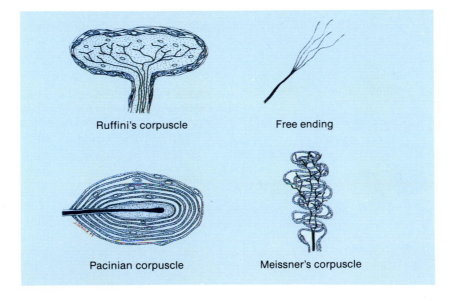

Figure 13.13 *Types of nerve endings found in the temporomandibular joint. The four types are* **Ruffini's,** *or temperature endings; the* **Pacinian,** *which is a pressure receptor,* **free** *nerve endings, which are pain endings; and* **Meissner's,** *which are touch receptors. These are represenative of the variety of receptors found in the capsule, disc, and soft tissues of the joint.*

Muscles of Mastication

There are eight powerful muscles of mastication—four on each side. Each has a different location; therefore, the direction of fiber contraction results in a different functional relationship. Three of the muscles on each side—the medial pterygoid, the masseter, and the temporalis—exert vertical forces in closing of the jaws, whereas the lateral pterygoid muscles function to protract the mandible and stabilize the joint. These muscles do not function alone but work as a group with the muscles of the tongue and the superhyoid muscles. **Free movements** of the mandible relate to the interplay of masticatory muscles and the morphology of the teeth without food, whereas **masticatory movement** is the synergistic action of the three groups of muscles—the elevators, depressors, and protractors that function together and at different times during mastication of food.

1. The **medial pterygoid** arises from the medial surface of the lateral pterygoid plate and inserts in the inferior surface of the ramus and angle of the mandible. Its blood supply is from the maxillary artery, and its nerve supply is from the mandibular division of the trigeminal artery. It functions to protract and elevate the mandible (Figure 13.14). The medial part runs down and backward, below and behind the angle of the mandible to meet the externally located masseter in a tendinous raphe and form the pterygomasseteric sling. (Figures 13.14 and 13.15).

2. The **lateral pterygoid** has two heads—the upper arising from the greater wing of the sphenoid and the lower from the lateral pterygoid plate. They insert into the front of the neck of the condyle and the capsule (Figure 13.15). The blood supply is from the maxillary artery, and the nerve supply is from the pterygoid branch of the mandibular artery. Both heads of this muscle function to protrude the mandible and pull the articular disc forward (Figures 13.14 and 13.15).

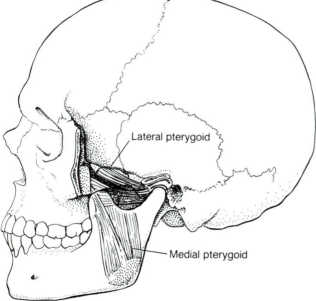

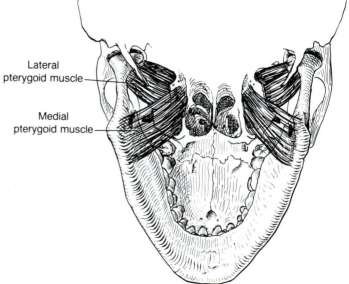

Figure 13.14 *The lateral and medial pterygoid muscles of mastication. The medial pterygoid functions in elevation and protraction of the joint. The lateral pterygoid functions to protrude the mandible and pull the articular disc anteriorly.*

Figure 13.15 *Inferior view of the medial and lateral pterygoids to illustrate their attachments to the mandible and base of the skull.*

3. The **temporalis** fibers originate from the floor of the temporal fossa and temporal fascia and insert on the anterior border of the coronoid process and anterior border of the ramus of the mandible (Figure 13.16). The blood supply is from the superficial temporal and maxillary arteries, and the nerve supply is from the deep temporal branches of the mandibular nerve. The functions of the temporalis muscle are elevation of the jaw, retraction of the mandible, and clenching of the teeth.

4. The **masseter** muscle has a deep part and superficial part. The superficial fibers originate from the anterior two thirds of the lower border of the zygomatic arch and the deep fibers from the medial surface of the same arch. The superficial fibers are at right angles to the occlusal plane of the posterior teeth, and the deep fibers are directed down and slightly anteriorly. This muscle inserts into the lateral

surface of the coronoid process of the mandible, the upper half of the ramus, and the angle of the mandible. The blood supply is from the superficial temporal and maxillary arteries, and the nerve supply comes from the mandibular division of the trigeminal nerve. The masseter muscle functions to elevate the jaw and clench the teeth (Figure 13.17).

■ *Clinical Comment*

A functional relationship of the occlusion of the teeth is expressed through the muscles of mastication. A detailed history and physical examination provide for an accurate diagnosis. Clinicians must rely on their own judgment in the treatment of patients with TMJ pain.

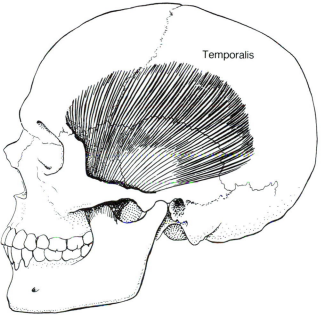

Figure 13.16 *The temporalis muscle of mastication. The temporalis muscle functions in elevation of the jaw, retraction of the mandible, and clenching of the teeth.*

Figure 13.17 *The masseter muscle of mastication. The function of the masseter muscle is to elevate the jaw and clench the teeth.*

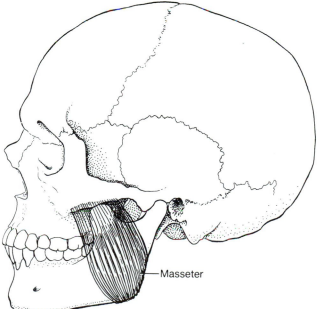

■ *Remodeling of TMJ Articulation*

Articular remodeling is the morphologic adaptation of the joint in response to environmental stress. The articular surfaces of the TMJ have been shown to adapt to minimize the effects of the stressful mandibular function. Presence of cartilage in the condyle and the articular disc allows the TMJ to withstand stress to a better extent than other fibrous joints. Progressive remodeling occurs when there is proliferation of the articular cartilage and production of intercellular matrix followed by its mineralization, then its resorption, and eventually replacement by bone (Figure 13.18). This may happen in one or both of the condylar heads and the articular eminences and may relate to any changes in structure of the articular surfaces. In some cases, remodeling may begin in the proliferation zone, causing an outgrowth of cartilage on the surface, which then becomes mineralized and replaced by bone at the zone of resorption. Functional adaptation is the response of chondrogenesis and osteogenesis to withstand the effects of compression and loading. In aging, with decreased cell proliferation, these changes may be degenerative.

■ *Clinical Comment*

Myofacial pain dysfunction, or *MPD,* continues to be an area of disagreement in clinical treatment. Since there is still much to be learned about both the normal and abnormal functions of the TMJ, more progress in the treatment of MPD can be expected.

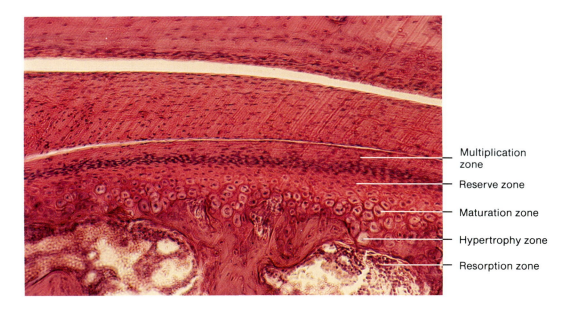

Multiplication zone

Reserve zone

Maturation zone

Hypertrophy zone

Resorption zone

Figure 13.18   *This histologic view of the head of the condyle illustrates the areas of response initiated in the reserve cartilage zone and ultimately stimulating the zone of bone replacement.*

■ Self-Evaluation Questions

1. What are the three supporting ligaments of the TMJ?
2. What is the role of the TMJ capsule?
3. Describe the two different functions in the lower and upper compartments of the TMJ.
4. How do the heads of the condyles change as a person grows and matures?
5. What are the functions of the two heads of the lateral pterygoid muscle?
6. What is meant by the sling muscles, and do they function similarly?
7. What is the function of the temporalis muscle?
8. What is the significance of the same innervation being supplied to both the TMJ and its respective muscles?
9. What is the blood supply to the TMJ?
10. What are synovial cells and their function?

■ Acknowledgments

Figures 13. 1 and 13.6 provided by Dr. D.W. Wright; 13.8 provided by Dr. C.C. Boyer; 13.2 and 13.18 provided by the now deceased Dr. S. Bernick. In Oral Development and Histology, Toronto, B.C. Decker, 1988.

■ Suggested Reading

Griffin, C.J., Hawthorne, R., and Harris, R. Anatomy and histology of the human temporomandibular joint. Monogr. Oral Sci. 1975; 4:1.

Karakasis, D., and Tsaknakis, A. Aging changes in the articular disk of the temporomandibular joint in the guinea pig. J. Dent. Res. 1976; 55:262.

Meikie, M.C. The role of condyle in the postnatal growth of the mandible. Am. J. Orthod. 1973; 64:50.

Sarnat, B.G., and Laskin, D.M. Temporomandibular joint: Biological basis for clinical practice. Springfield, Ill.: Charles C Thomas, 1979.

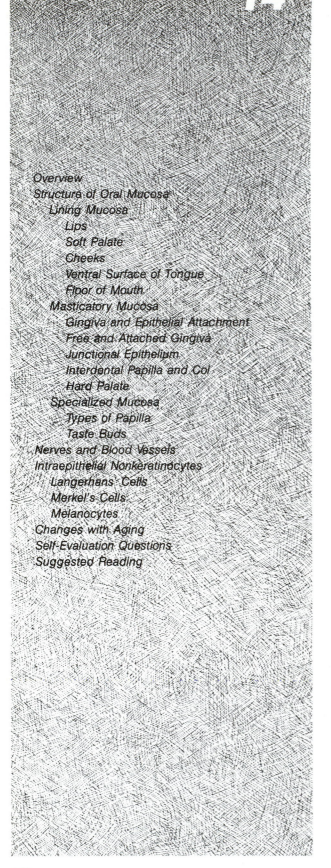

Oral Mucosa

■ Overview

The structure of stratified squamous epithelium of the oral mucosa varies from the nonkeratinized lining mucosa of the cheeks, lips, soft palate, and floor of the mouth to the keratinized epithelium covering the palate and alveolar ridges. The masticatory mucosa consists of multiple layers of epithelial cells located on the dermis or lamina propria layer, which contains serous, mucous, or mixed glands, blood vessels, and nerve endings. A third type of mucosa, found on the surface of the tongue, is specialized mucosa. It consists of four types of papillae: filiform, fungiform, foliate, and circumvallate.

Taste is associated with the latter three types of papillae, which are located on the tongue as well as the soft palate and pharynx. Four types of taste are regionally associated with the tongue. At the tip, sweet and salty tastes are perceived, sour taste is associated with the sides of the tongue, and bitter taste at the back of the tongue.

Masticatory mucosa includes the gingiva, which is composed of the tissue surrounding the necks of the teeth. The gingiva consists of three areas: free, attached, and interdental. The free gingiva is characterized by the gingival sulcus. The attached gingiva has junctional epithelium, which binds the gingiva to the necks of the teeth. The interdental area is that tissue between teeth below their contact point. The hard palate is also covered by masticatory mucosa, which is firmly attached to the underlying bone.

Cells of the oral mucosa are termed keratinocytes and can be distinguished from the nonkeratinocytes, which are Langerhans' cells, Merkel's cells, and melanocytes. In case of inflammation, lymphocytes and leukocytes may appear in the mucosa. They are commonly found in gingival epithelium.

Four types of nerve receptors—heat, cold, pain, and touch—are located in the lips and oral cavity. They are most numerous in the lips and tip of the tongue. With age, the oral mucosa becomes thinner and may be located lower on the necks of teeth. It may be less moist because of the decrease in activity of the salivary glands.

■ *Structure of Oral Mucosa*

The oral cavity is lined with stratified squamous epithelium, which is divided into three types of different tissue. **Lining mucosa** covers the floor of the mouth and lines the cheeks, lips, and soft palate. It does not function in mastication and therefore has little attrition. **Masticatory mucosa** covers the palate and alveolar ridges and is so termed because it comes in primary contact with food during mastication. **Specialized mucosa,** which covers the surface of the tongue, is quite different in structure and appearance from the two previous tissues.

Each type of tissue has structural differences: the lining mucosa is soft, pliable, and nonkeratinized; the masticatory mucosa is keratinized, indicative of the attrition that takes place during mastication; the specialized mucosa on the tongue surface is covered largely with cornified epithelial papillae, which function in mastication. The mucosa of the oral cavity has several features common to epithelium elsewhere in the body. One of these features is the lamina propria. This is the connective tissue layer immediately below the epithelium. It is composed of the papillary and deeper reticular layer (Figure 14.1). In the papillary layer, the connective tissue extends into pockets in the epithelium. This increases the surface of the epithelium for contact with vascular supply and nerves. The reticular layer contains the deeper plexi of vessels and nerves supported by connective tissue. These two layers, papillary and reticular, contribute the lamina propria or dermis. Beneath this zone is the submucosa or subcutaneous tissue.

Lining Mucosa

Lining mucosa extends in depth from the underlying dermis to the free surface of the cheeks and floor of the mouth. It is composed of a basal cell layer of cuboidal cells, termed the **stratum basale.** The next several cell layers are called the **stratum intermedium** or **stratum spinosum.** The cells in this layer appear oval and somewhat flattened. The third, or superficial, layer is termed the **stratum superficiale.** Its cells are flattened, and many contain small oval nuclei (Figure 14.1). These three cell layers form the non-keratinized epithelium of the oral mucosa and appear similar to the epithelium in the pharynx. The other component of the mucosa is the dermis, composed of the papillary and reticulum connective tissue layers.

The characteristics of lining mucosa in each area follow.

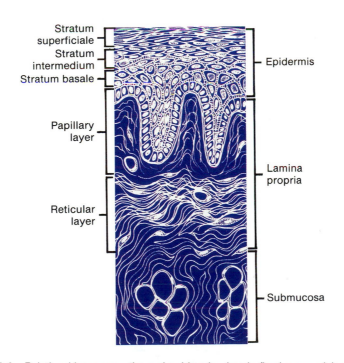

Figure 14.1 *Relationships among the oral epidermis, dermis (lamina propria), and submucosal tissue. The names of the layers of the epidermis and dermis are noted on the left.*

Lips

The inner oral surface of the lips is lined with moist-surface, stratified squamous, nonkeratinized epithelium, which is associated with small, round seromucous glands of the lamina propria. These glands are part of the minor salivary glands found throughout the oral cavity. Beneath the dermis is the submucosa, in which fibers of the orbicularis oris muscle are located (Figure 14.2). Nonkeratinized mucosa of the lips is distinguished by a red border known as the **vermilion border.** This area is at the junction between the oral mucosa and the skin of the lips, which becomes modified into keratinized epithelium different from skin or mucosa. There are three reasons why the vermilion border is red: epithelium is thin; this epithelium contains **eleidin,** which is transparent; and the blood vessels are close to the surface of the papillary layer, revealing the red blood cells' color (Figure 14.3). Also observable in the skin of the lips are hair follicles and their associated sebaceous glands, erector pili muscles, and sweat glands. Sebaceous glands can be seen at the angles of the mouth. They are not associated with hair follicles. These glands are known as **Fordyce's spots** (Figure 14.4).

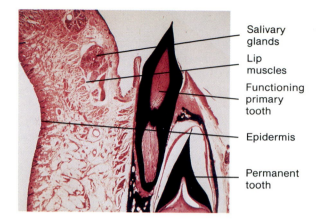

Figure 14.2 *Histology of the lip and alveolar bone, which contains a functioning primary and developing permanent tooth.*

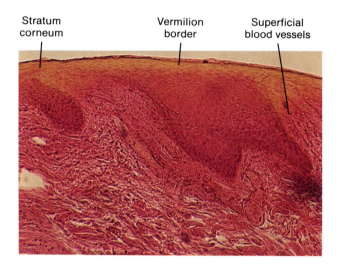

Figure 14.3 *Vermilion border of the lip illustrating the thin and lucent stratum corneum and the presence of capillaries in the papillary layer. Observe the close relationship of the blood supply to the surface of the vermilion border epithelium.*

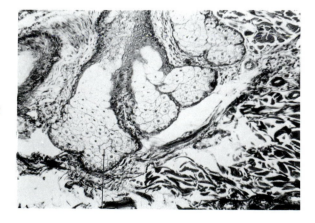

Figure 14.4 *Fordyce's spots, sebaceous glands not related to hair follicles, are found at the angles of the mouth.*

Soft Palate

Lining mucosa of the highly vascularized soft palate is more pink than the mucosa of the keratinized epithelium of the hard palate (Figure 14.5). This tissue is pink, since the **lamina propria** contains many small blood vessels. Beneath the connective tissue of the lamina propria is the submucosa, which contains muscles of the soft palate and mucous glands.

Cheeks

The mucosa of the cheeks is like that of the lips or soft palate since each has nonkeratinized stratified squamous epithelium, lamina propria, and underlying submucosa. In the cheeks, however, the submucosa contains fat cells and mixed glands (seromucous) located within and between the muscle fibers of the cheeks. The presence of these glands and fat cells is a unique feature of the cheeks (Figure 14.6).

■ **Clinical Comment**

Observing change in a patient's oral mucosa is based in part on recognition of the individual's normal characteristics and on evaluation of the patient's history. Among the basic conditions of the mucosa to be considered are variations in tissue color, dryness, smoothness, or firmness, and whether the gingiva bleeds easily. Saliva should be normal in amount and consistency.

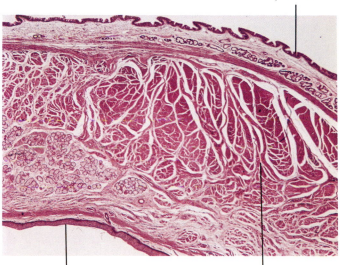

Figure 14.5 *Section cut in the sagittal plane of the soft palate (anterior on the left). The nasal cavity is above, and respiratory epithelium covers the superior part of the soft palate. The oral cavity below is covered with squamous epithelium. Observe the glands underlying the oral mucosa and muscle throughout the submucosa.*

Pharyngeal epithelium

Oral epithelium — Seromucous glands between muscle fibers — Muscles of soft palate

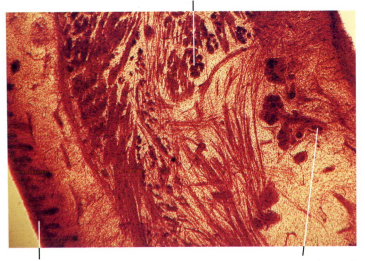

Figure 14.6 *Histology of the tissues of cheek. Skin is seen on the left and oral mucosa on the right. Observe the glands intermingled with the muscle fibers in the subcutaneous zone of the cheek.*

Skin

Duct of gland to oral mucosal surface

Ventral Surface of Tongue

This lining mucosa also contains a lamina propria and submucosa. In the submucosa, muscle fibers are located under the surface of the tongue. The entire area exhibits dense, interlaced muscle and connective tissue fibers. Limits of the submucosa are not distinct since the submucosa continues with the deep muscles of the tongue along with connective tissue fibers (Figure 14.7).

Floor of Mouth

Nonkeratinized mucous membrane covers the floor of the mouth and appears loosely attached to the underlying dermis as compared to the adjacent tongue mucosa. (Compare Figures 14.7 and 14.8). In the floor of the mouth are found minor salivary glands (Figure 14.8) and the major mucous gland, the **sublingual gland.**

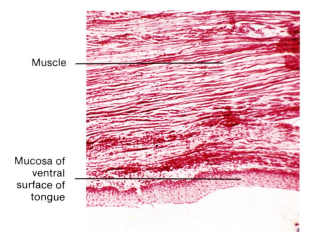

Muscle

Mucosa of ventral surface of tongue

Figure 14.7 *Histology of the ventral surface of the tongue. Observe the density of the muscle fibers intermingling in the dermis.*

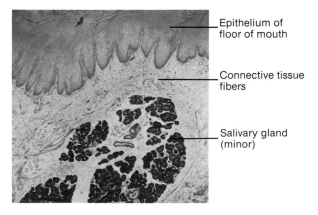

Epithelium of floor of mouth

Connective tissue fibers

Salivary gland (minor)

Figure 14.8 *Histology of the lining mucosa of the floor of the mouth. Observe the lack of muscle fibers and the delicate appearance of the connective tissue fibers. Scattered islands of minor serous and mucous salivary glands are seen near the tip of the tongue.*

Masticatory Mucosa

Masticatory mucosa is epithelium covering the gingiva and hard palate. This mucosa is thicker than the nonkeratinized mucosa with the addition of a keratinized surface of flat, hornified cells offering resistance to attrition. The basal and intermediate stratum **(stratum spinosum)** layers are the same as those of nonkeratinized epithelium. There are two other layers, the granular layer, or **stratum granulosum,** and the surface layer, or **stratum corneum** (Figure 14.9). The cells of the basal layer are cuboidal or columnar, and their nuclei are irregularly oval and exhibit numerous mitotic figures as they undergo constant cell division. These cells then migrate from the basal layer to the surface of the mucosa. Figure 14.9 is useful in describing the differences in each cell layer. The second layer, or stratum spinosum, is several cells thick. These cells are oval to polygonal, and mitotic figures can also be seen in this layer. Basal cells interface with a membrane separating the epithelium and connective tissue. This membrane is termed the **basal lamina** (Figure 14.10). The basal cells are attached to the basal lamina by minute discs, termed hemidesmosomes (Figure 14.10). These thickenings of the cell membrane are supported by filaments from within the cells, anchoring fibrils attaching the basal lamina and the epithelial cells to the collagen fibers of the dermis. These structures are seen in Figure 14.11.

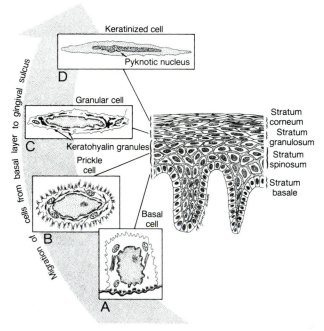

Figure 14.9 *The keratinized stratified squamous epithelium of the oral cavity. Observe the characteristics of the four cell types of this epithelium, from the basal to the surface layers.*

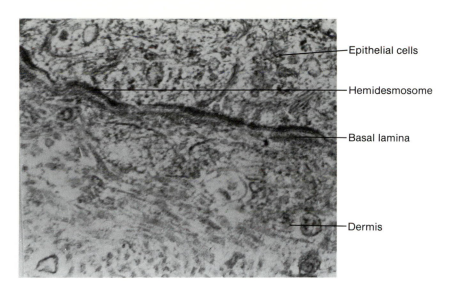

Figure 14.10 *Ultrastructure of the junction of the epithelium and dermis as seen in this electron micrograph. The basal lamina extends across the field from left to right, to which the epithelial cells are attached by hemidesmosomes.*

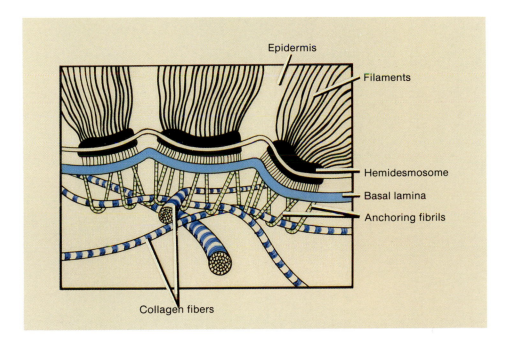

Figure 14.11 *Diagram of hemidesmosomes of the oral mucosa. Observe the basal lamina, and observe how the hemidesmosomes of the epithelial cells attach to this membrane. Collagen fibers of the connective tissue attach to the fibers of the hemidesmosome.*

All epithelial cells exhibit intracellular filaments, **tonofibrils,** that project to the cell surface and attach to **desmosomes** (Figures 14.11 and 14.12). Desmosomes are cell-to-cell junctions, which in oral mucosa are discoid and called **macula adherens.** These junctions are composed of several thin protein adhesion discs located between the cells. These discs temporarily hold the cells in contact. Later, these junctions release the cells so that they can migrate more superficially and reattach with other desmosomes in a new location. The stratum spinosum cells may also exhibit a few keratohyalin granules.

The next layer of cells superficially is the stratum granulosum, so named because the cells contain many keratinohyalin granules (Figure 14.13). The surface layer of cells, the stratum corneum, is characterized by thin, flattened, non-nucleated cells. These cells are filled with a soft keratin that replaces the cell cytoplasm. This soft keratin may be compared to the hard keratin of the nails and hair. Keratin is tough, nonliving material resistant to friction and impervious to bacterial invasion.

To permit cell movement and loss of individual cells along the surface, the superficial layers have surface interdigitations rather than desmosomes. These cells are continually becoming lost and replaced by cells of the underlying layers.

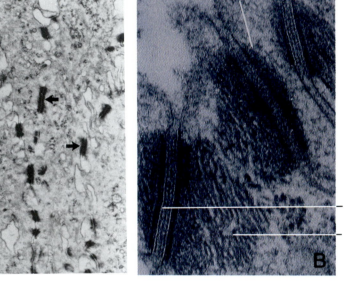

A

B

— Desmosome

— Tonofibrils

Figure 14.12 *Histology (electron micrograph) of cell junctions of the oral epithelial cells. These are termed desmosomes. (A) In low power, arrows indicate the button-like attachments between each cell. (B) At higher magnification, is the multilayer arrangement of the desmosomes. Note that tonofibrils of the cell attach to these plate-like cell junctions.*

Figure 14.13 *Histology of the oral epithelium. This is an electron micrograph of keratinized oral epithelium. Observe the relative thickness of each cell layer from stratum basale to stratum corneum and the lamina propria beneath the epithelium.*

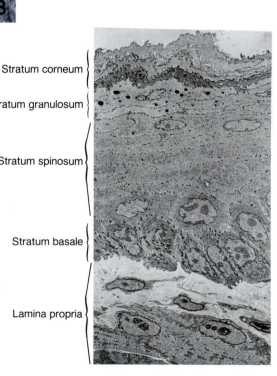

Stratum corneum

Stratum granulosum

Stratum spinosum

Stratum basale

Lamina propria

Gingiva and Epithelial Attachment

In the oral mucosa, the gingiva surrounds the necks of the teeth and extends apically to the mucogingival junction (Figure 14.14). The gingiva develops as a coalescence of the oral and reduced enamel organ epithelia when the tooth first emerges in the oral cavity (Figure 14.15 *A* to *C*). The reduced enamel organ epithelium contacts the undersurface of the oral epithelium and the two fuse. Then the tooth penetrates this combined layer to enter the mouth and produces the gingiva (a cuff of epithelium) as the epithelium continues to separate from the enamel surface until occlusion of the teeth is reached (Figure 14.15*C*). At this point, the gingiva covers only the cervical area of the enamel where it is attached (Figure 14.15*D*).

The gingiva is divided into three zones: (1) the **free or marginal zone,** which encircles the tooth and defines the gingival sulcus; (2) the **attached gingiva,** that portion of the epithelium attached to the neck of the tooth by means of **junctional epithelium;** (3) and the **interdental zone** (groove), the area between two adjacent teeth beneath their contact point (Figure 14.14). The free and attached gingiva may have an indistinct groove on the surface of the epithelium separating them. This groove is termed the **free gingival groove** (Figures 14.14 and 14.16).

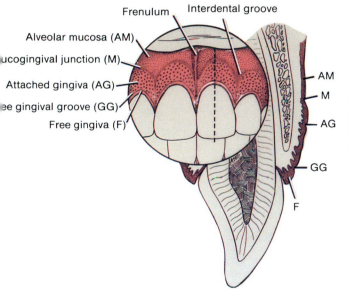

Figure 14.14 *The gingiva shown in both facial and longitudinal views. Observe the free gingiva (F) along the crest of the gingiva, the stippled attached gingiva (AG), and the mucogingival groove (M), which separates the gingiva from the alveolar mucosa. Note also the frenulum and interdental zones (grooves).*

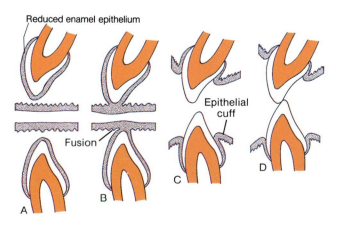

Figure 14.15 *(A to D) The gingiva develops from the reduced enamel epithelium of the tooth and the oral epithelium. The two meet, fuse, and then rupture to allow the tooth to erupt.*

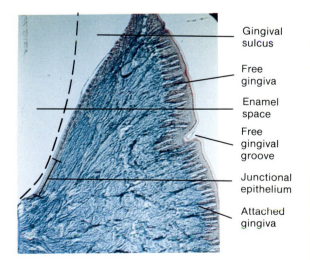

Figure 14.16 *Histology of the gingiva illustrating the gingival sulcus, the junctional epithelium, and the free gingiva. The enamel space is created by loss (decalcification) of the enamel.*

Free and Attached Gingiva

The free or marginal gingiva is bound on its inner margin by the gingival sulcus, which separates it from the tooth; on its outer margin by the oral cavity; and apically at its free surface by the **free gingival groove** (Figure 14.17). This groove separates the free from the attached gingiva. Therefore, the attached gingiva lies adjacent to the free gingiva and is separated from the alveolar mucosa by the **mucogingival junction** (Figure 14.17). The free and attached gingiva are keratinized, but the alveolar mucosa is not. The attached gingiva is stippled, but the free gingiva has a smooth surface (Figure 14.18). In some instances the free gingiva may be covered with parakeratinized mucosa, which are keratinized cells modified by the presence of nuclei in the cells of the surface layer. The unique feature of attached gingiva is the junctional epithelium.

Junctional Epithelium

Junctional epithelium provides the attachment of the gingiva to the tooth in the cervical area and forms the epithelial-lined floor of the gingival sulcus (Figure 14.19). The cells of the attached epithelium are cytologically different from other cells of the gingival epithelium. They have fewer desmosomes (cell attachment buttons), which indicates a higher rate of turnover than with other gingival epithelial cells (Figure 14.19). These cells have been reported to turn over in approximately six days from the time of their appearance in the stratum basale to that in the surface where they are sloughed. These cells also have many organelles: rough endoplasmic reticulum, Golgi's apparatus, and mitochondria, indicating high metabolic activity.

The stratum basale cells also contain **hemidesmosomes,** the mechanism of attachment for these cells to a salivary protein layer covering the cervical area of the enamel (Figure 14.20). These cells are actually half a desmosome and are the same type of structure with which the basal cells of squamous epithelium interface and attach to the basal lamina and connective tissue of the gingiva (see Figure 14.12). Disturbance of this attachment to the tooth by infection, food impaction, calculus, or other irritants results in a deepening of the gingival sulcus.

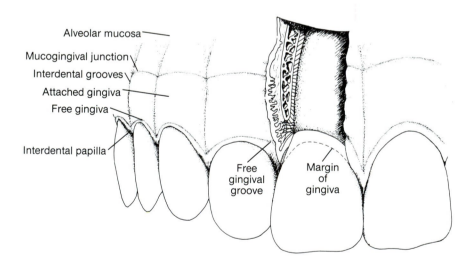

Alveolar mucosa

Mucogingival junction

Interdental grooves

Attached gingiva

Free gingiva

Interdental papilla

Free gingival groove

Margin of gingiva

Figure 14.17 *The location of the free and attached gingiva and the location of the mucogingival junction, which separates the keratinized gingiva from the nonkeratinized alveolar mucosa.*

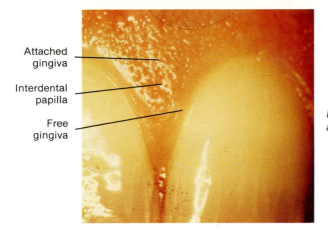

Attached gingiva

Interdental papilla

Free gingiva

Figure 14.18 *A view of normal gingiva illustrating the free and attached (stippled) gingiva.*

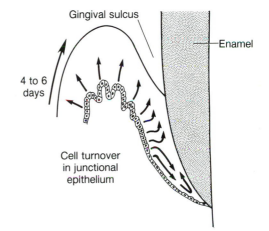

Gingival sulcus

Enamel

4 to 6 days

Cell turnover in junctional epithelium

Figure 14.19 *Epithelial cell turnover in the gingiva. Note the direction of epithelial cell maturation from basal cell to surface in the attachment zone and at the margin of the gingiva.*

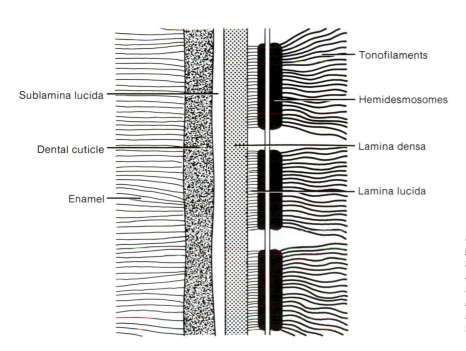

Tonofilaments

Sublamina lucida

Hemidesmosomes

Dental cuticle

Lamina densa

Lamina lucida

Enamel

Figure 14.20 *The means of gingival attachment with the tooth's surface. The hemidesmosome is a specialized attachment plaque that attaches to the protein (cuticle or pellicle) on the tooth's surface. If the hemidesmosome is disturbed, reattachment may take place.*

Interdental Papilla and Col

Gingiva located between the teeth extending high on the interproximal area of the crowns on the labial and lingual surfaces is known as the **interdental papillae** (see Figure 14.18). This tissue fills the space created by the constricted cervical regions of the adjacent crowns. In the interproximal area, between the vestibular and lingual papillae, is a concave zone of gingiva that follows the contour of each crown (Fig. 14.21). When the gingiva is inflamed or hyperemic, the **col** is exaggerated and is positioned higher on the tooth (Fig. 14.22). The col is characterized as a thin, non-keratinized epithelium, whose basal epithelial cells invade the connective tissue where inflammatory cells of the lamina propria may appear (Fig. 14.23). The col is more inclined in a peak anteriorly and becomes more flattened between the posterior teeth.

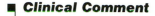

■ *Clinical Comment*

In examining the gingiva, one should keep in mind its normal appearance as discussed in this chapter. From this viewpoint, other than normal conditions can be more easily recognized.

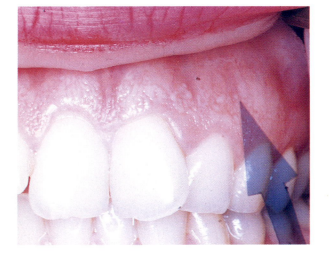

Figure 14.21 *Clinical view of the gingiva showing the free and attached gingiva and an interdental groove (arrow). The col is found in this area.*

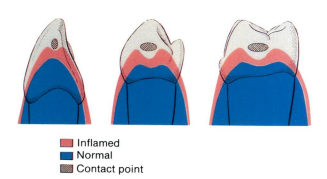

- 🟥 Inflamed
- 🟦 Normal
- ▨ Contact point

Figure 14.22 *The positional relationship of the col in health and disease. Note the col is accentuated in inflammation and swelling of the gingiva. Observe that the col is pointed anteriorly and flat to concave posteriorly.*

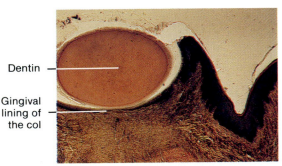

Dentin —

Gingival lining of the col —

Figure 14.23 *Histology of the col, the concave non-keratinized epithelial lining of the gingiva between the teeth. The contact point is represented by the dentin seen above the col.*

Hard Palate

The roof of the mouth, or hard palate, is covered with keratinized stratified squamous epithelium. This epithelium is similar to that of the gingiva in the midline area where there is no submucosa. The midline is known as the **median raphe,** which may only be fairly discernible, except anteriorly where an incisive papilla may be seen. On each side of the median raphe are ridges of tissue called **rugae** (Figure 14.24). These folds of epithelium are supported by dense lamina propria (Figure 14.25). In the anterior lateral palate, there is a zone of fatty tissue located in the submucosa, and in the posterior hard palate, there is mucous glandular tissue (see Figure 14.24). Both the hard and soft palates have mucous glands. **Traction bands** (Figure 14.26) exist in the dermis of the rugae between the lobules of fatty tissue and the glands of the anterior and posterior hard palate. These bands are bundles of collagen fibers that insert into the papillary fibers of the lamina propria and extend into the bony palate. They anchor the palatal mucosa to the underlying bone. The hard palate assists in mastication.

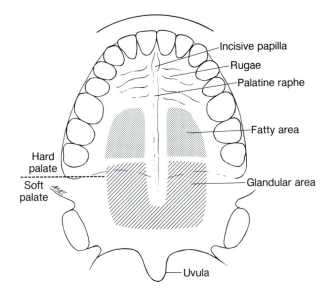

Figure 14.24   *The palate. After noting the landmarks, observe the location of the glandular zone anteriorly and the fatty zone posteriorly in the subcutaneous zone. There is no subcutaneous tissue, only dermis in the midline and in the gingival area.*

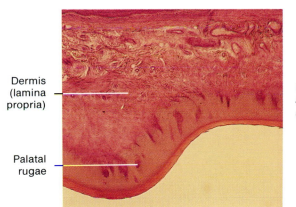

Dermis (lamina propria)

Palatal rugae

Figure 14.25   *Histologic section in the anterior palate showing the rugae. Rugae are epithelial-covered folds in the dermis in the anterior area of the palate.*

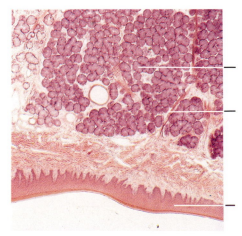

Glandular tissue

Traction band

Palatal mucosa

Figure 14.26   *Histologic section of the palate in the glandular zone. Traction bands of collagen fibers bind the palatal epithelium to the underlying bone.*

Specialized Mucosa

Types of Papillae

The dorsum or superior surface of the tongue (anterior two thirds) is covered with a specialized mucosa. This mucosa consists of four types of epithelial structures called **papillae** (Figure 14.27). The **filiform papillae** are slender, thread-like keratinized extensions of the surface epithelial cells. Interspersed with the filiform papillae are a few **fungiform papillae,** which are more numerous toward the tip of the tongue (Figure 14.27). The roughened surface of the tongue is provided by the 2 to 3 mm high filiform papilla (Figures 14.28 and 14.29). They facilitate movement of food in the mouth. The fungiform papillae are shaped like a mushroom, with the cap sometimes larger than the stalk (Figure 14.30). The covering epithelium is thin, so it appears pink or reddish in the mouth because blood vessels are near the surface (Figure 14.30). Taste buds are occa-

sionally found on the superior surface of the fungiform papillae (Figures 14.30 and 14.31B). A third type of papilla is the **circumvallate papillae,** which are only 10 to 14 in number and located along the V-shaped sulcus between the body and base of the tongue (Figures 14.31A and B). These papillae are level with the surface of the tongue, and each has a surrounding groove. They are large—3 mm in diameter.

Ducts of the underlying serous glands (von Ebner's) are seen opening into the grooves surrounding the papillae, and taste buds line the walls of the papillae (Figure 14.31B). The watery secretion of these glands washes out these trenches so that new tastes can be perceived. On the lateral and posterior sides of the tongue are vertical grooves or furrows, which also contain taste buds (see Figure 14.31A). These are called **foliate papillae.** Like circumvallate papillae, they contain taste buds, and the watery section of serous glands cleanses the grooves of these papillae (Figure 14.31B).

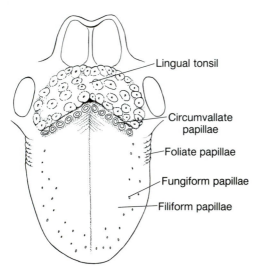

Figure 14.27 *The dorsal surface of the tongue showing the papillae on the tongue. The filiform papillae are scattered over the surface of the body of the tongue. The fungiform papillae are large, round, and pink and occur occasionally in this area. The foliate papillae are 4 to 11 in number and appear on the posterolateral aspect of the tongue. There are 8 to 10 circumvallate papillae located at the junction of the body and the base (tonsillar area) of the tongue.*

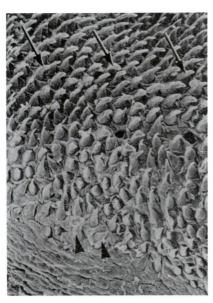

Figure 14.28 *A scanning electron micrograph of filiform papillae (arrows). These pointed papillae point toward the throat and assist in moving food in that direction as the tongue moves.*

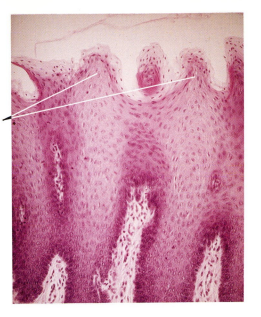

Filiform
papillae

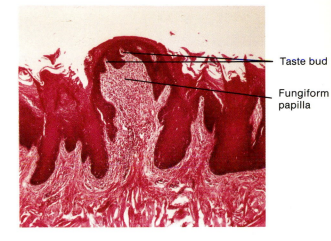

Taste bud

Fungiform
papilla

Figure 14.30 *Histologic section of a fungiform papilla with a connective tissue core and epithelial covering. Two taste buds are located on the dorsal surface of this papilla.*

Figure 14.29 *A histologic picture of the filiform papillae of the dorsal surface of the tongue. Note these pointed keratinized projections.*

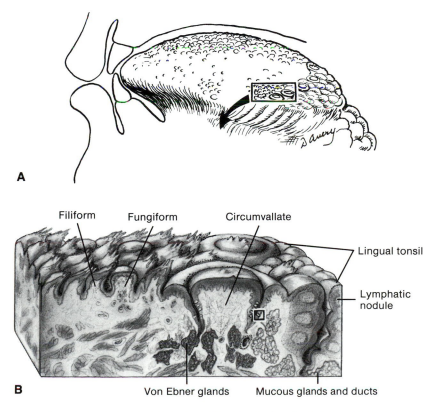

A

Filiform   Fungiform   Circumvallate

Lingual tonsil

Lymphatic
nodule

B

Von Ebner glands   Mucous glands and ducts

Figure 14.31 *(A) Circumvallate papillae. Note the large 2-mm papillae with a trench around each and the underlying serous (von Ebner's) glands, which wash out the taste from the area of the taste buds. (B) Dorsal appearance of the tongue with fungiform, filiform, and circumvallate papillae. A taste bud is shown within the small rectangular area.*

Taste Buds

The taste buds are small barrel-shaped bodies. These discrete sense organs contain the chemical sense of taste. They are generally associated with the papillae previously described, although some are distributed on the soft palate, epiglottis, larynx, and pharynx (see Figures 14.32 to 14.34 and Table 14.1).

Taste buds are easily recognized under the microscope as barrel-shaped structures; their epithelial cells appear ovoid (Figure 14.34). Although they have been referred to as neuroepithelial structures, they are more correctly referred to as epithelial cells with club-shaped sensory nerve endings arising from the chorda tympani that come to lie among the taste cells.

There are several types of cells in a taste bud: **taste cells,** usually 10 to 14 in each taste bud; **supporting** or sustentacular cells (several types) that lie in the periphery of the taste bud; and **basal cells,** which are perpendicular to the basal lamina and believed to be a stem cell for the other two types of cells (Figure 14.34). There is a rapid turnover of these cells, approximately 10 days.

Four types of taste sensations can be detected, and there is evidence of regional sensitivity for these tastes on the tongue and palate. The four taste sensations are: sweet, salty, sour, and bitter. Sensations of **sweet** and **salty** are perceived at the tongue's tip, **sour** on the sides, and **bitter** in the region of the circumvallate papillae (Figure 14.35). These areas overlap, and evidence indicates that all papillae may respond to all four types of taste sensations. However, the levels of sensitivity differ. For example, with higher concentrations of a bitter taste, the sensation is perceived most notably on the posterior segment of the tongue. This indicates a regional selectivity of taste in the mouth which may be due in part to the origin of the nerve supply.

Nerves for taste buds of the anterior two thirds of the tongue pass to the chorda tympani branch of the facial nerve, those of the posterior one third pass to the glossopharyngeal nerve, and those from the epiglottis and pharynx pass to the vagus nerve.

Mixing the four basic modalities of taste cannot explain all of the flavors that humans are capable of experiencing. Factors such as odor and temperature also contribute to flavors. In addition, taste buds can discriminate subtleties in flavor, such as the difference between citric or acetic acid. This enables taste buds to identify specific substances even when mixed.

Table 14.1 Location and Number of Taste Buds in the Human Adult

Tongue	10,000
Soft palate	2,500
Epiglottis	900
Larynx and pharynx	600
Oropharynx	250

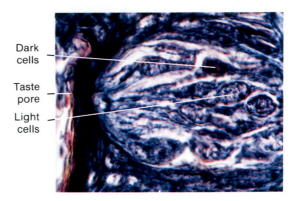

Figure 14.32 *Histology of a taste bud with its light and dark cells. The taste pore for reception of tasteable substances opens in the trench.*

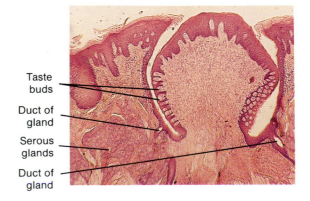

Figure 14.33 *Histology of a circumvallate papilla with taste buds located on its walls in the trench. Note the gland and its duct emptying into the trench from the lower left and right.*

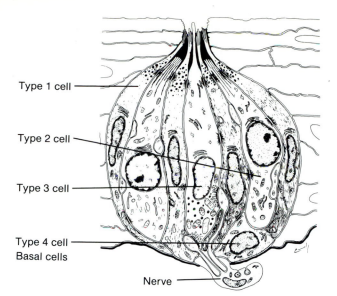

Type 1 cell

Type 2 cell

Type 3 cell

Type 4 cell
Basal cells

Nerve

Figure 14.34 *A typical taste bud. Four types of cells are noted. Type 1 dark cells represent 60 percent of the cells; type 2 light cells represent 30 percent; and type 3, 7 percent. Type 4, the basal cells, represent 3 percent.*

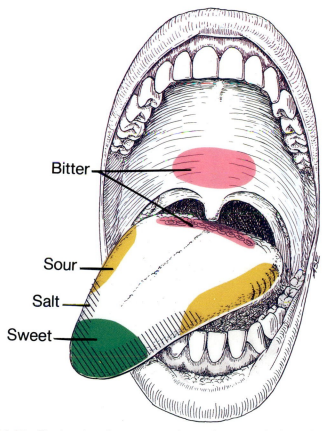

Bitter

Sour

Salt

Sweet

Figure 14.35 *The location of taste perception on the tongue in the oral cavity. The tip has sweet receptors, along the front sides are salty receptors, on the posterior sides are sour receptors, and in the posterior center and soft palate are bitter receptors.*

■ Nerves and Blood Vessels

The nerves and blood vessels of the gingiva appear in the lamina propria. Terminal endings of nerves and loops of blood vessels appear in the dermal papillae. There blood vessels consist of a deep plexus of larger vessels in the submucosa underlying the lamina propria, and capillary loops extend into a secondary plexus in the dermal papillae. The epithelium is avascular, and its metabolic needs must come from the vessels of the lamina propria. Nutrition passes from these vessels through the connective tissue and basal lamina and then enters the epithelium. Throughout the gingiva, nerves and nerve endings are prevalent. The encapsulated touch and temperature endings are located in the papillary tissue of the lamina propria and anxons associated with Merkel's cells (Figure 14.36). Free endings associated with pain can be seen entering the epithelium between the cells (Figure 14.36). The areas and levels of sensitivity are seen in Table 14.2.

Table 14.2   Levels of Sensitivity of the Oral Region

Sensation	Greatest sensitivity	Moderate sensitivity
Pain	Lips, pharynx Base of tongue	Anterior tongue Gingiva
Heat	Lips	Tip of tongue
Cold	Lips, posterior palate	Base of tongue; ventral tongue
Touch	Lips, tip of tongue	Gingiva

■ Clinical Comment

The distribution of nerve endings in the oral cavity is greatest in the lips and anterior oral mucosa and least in the more posterior regions of the oral cavity. Therefore, the mouth tests food and beverages before they are taken farther into the alimentary canal. The one exception to this anterior sensitivity is that cold and pain nerve endings are numerous in the posterior palate.

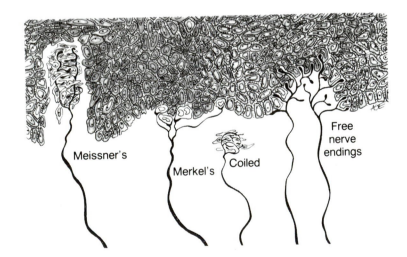

Figure 14.36   *The nerves in the oral mucosa showing the location of the various types of nerve endings within the oral mucosa.*

■ Intraepithelial Nonkeratinocytes

In contrast to the epithelial cells or keratinocytes, the non-keratinocytes make up about 10 percent of the mucosal cell population. These cells have a clear halo around their nuclei and have been called "clear cells." The three types of these cells are: **Langerhans' cells, Merkel's cells,** and **melanocytes.** There are two other nonkeratinocytes, which are lymphocytes and polymorphonuclear leukocytes that may also appear in the epithelium in case of inflammation.

Langerhans' Cells

Langerhans' cells are found in the stratum spinosum and are believed to function in the processing of antigenic material. They are therefore in an ideal location to contact invading bacteria and set up response mechanisms to protect the body. The cell appears to have processes but does not have desmosomes or tonofilaments. This cell has unique racket-shaped organelles (Figure 14.37A to C).

Merkel's Cells

Merkel's cells are located in the basal layer of the gingival epithelium. Unlike keratinocytes, they are associated with a terminal axon, and they contain round electron-dense granules in the cytoplasm adjacent to the axon. This cell and its axon are believed to function as a touch receptor (Figure 14.38).

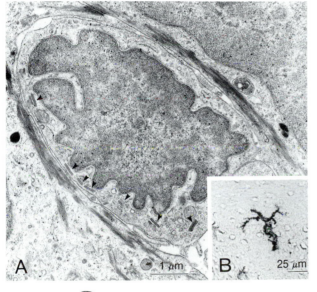

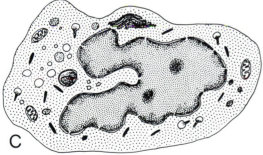

Figure 14.37 (A to C) Three histologic views of the non-keratinocytes, Langerhans' cells in the gingiva. They are large oval cells. Note the rodlike Langerhans granules in A.

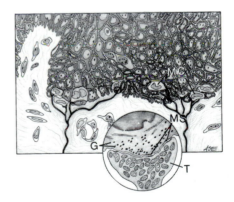

Figure 14.38 The Merkel's cells located in the basal cell layer and their relationship to a nerve ending (MS). The inset shows nerve terminals (T) with secretory granules (G) in Merkel's cell.

Melanocytes

Melanocytes are melanin-producing cells in the basal layer of the gingival epithelium. Melanocytes lack desmosomes and tonofilaments and are dendritic. A characteristic feature of the melanocyte is the melanin granules (melanosomes) found in the cytoplasm. Such cells may inject melanosomes into the nearby keratinocytes (Figure 14.39).

Lymphocytes, leukocytes, and mast cells, which are associated with gingival inflammation, may be found in the gingival epithelium and connective tissue. They may be located anywhere in the gingiva but most often underlie the junctional epithelium. Their appearance is different from that of keratinocytes owing to the absence of desmosomes, tonofilaments, and organelles. These lymphocytes appear typical, with a large oval nucleus occupying most of the cytoplasmic space.

■ *Changes with Aging*

Recognition of changes in the oral mucosa associated with aging is important. With age, the oral epithelium becomes thinner and more fragile. There is a flattening of the surface ridges and cells, and the oral mucosa appears smoother. Because of gradual atrophy of the minor salivary glands and less activity of the major glands, the oral mucosa has a drier appearance. In aging, there is decreased cellular activity, which relates to a general decrease in metabolic activity along with an increase in fibrosis, and the appearance of calcifications in the lamina propria of the gingiva and periodontal ligament. The ability to repair is reduced, and the length of healing time is increased. Apical migration of the gingiva is usually associated with disease but appears more routinely in the aging oral mucosa. Compare Figures 14.40 and 14.41.

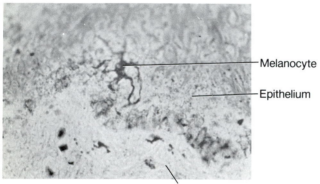

Figure 14.39 *Histology of another type of nonkeratinocyte. Note the location of the dendritic melanocyte in the stratum basale.*

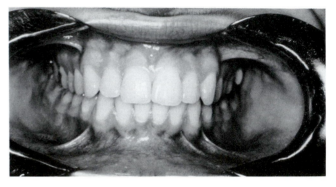

Figure 14.40 *Healthy gingiva in a 25-year-old shows normal color, form, and density.*

■ *Clinical Comment*

Halitosis can be due to multiple factors. If the ingestion of offensive foods is ruled out as a cause, possible food impaction, plaque, or the need for an oral prophylaxis should be considered. Disease of tooth origin or the periodontium could be another cause. Disease of the tonsils, disease of sinus origin, and systemic factors such as lung problems are also possible causes.

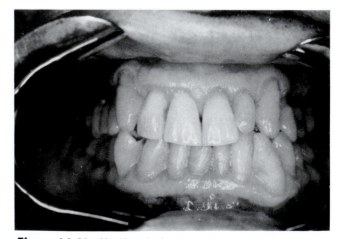

Figure 14.41 *Healthy gingiva in an 80-year-old differs from that in the 25-year-old in Figure 14.40 in that normal form and contours are altered.*

■ Self-Evaluation Questions

1. Define the several areas of the gingiva, and describe the characteristics of each.
2. Where are taste buds most numerous in the mouth?
3. List the three reasons lips are pink.
4. What is the function of the Langerhans' cells?
5. Name four types of nerve endings in the mouth, and state where each is in dense concentration.
6. Which appears more pink—the masticatory or lining mucosa—and why?
7. Name the types of papillae most numerous and least numerous on the tongue.
8. What are the locations and functions of traction bands?
9. What taste is recognized on the tip, lateral border, and more posterior region of the tongue?
10. What is the name of the sebaceous glands in the angle of the mouth?

■ Acknowledgments

Figure 14.10 provided by Dr. D. Turner, University of Michigan, School of Dentistry. Figure 14.13 provided by Dr. D. MacCullum, University of Michigan, School of Medicine. Figure 14.28 provided by Dr. M. Pirbazane. Figure 14.34 provided by Dr. R. Murray, Department of Anatomy, University of Indiana, School of Medicine. Figure 14.37 provided by Dr. I. Mackenzie, University of Iowa. Figures 14.40 and 14.41 provided by Dr. R. Courtney, University of Michigan, School of Dentistry.

■ Suggested Reading

Bhaskar, S.N. Orban's oral histology and embryology. St. Louis, C.V. Mosby, 1986.

Gibaldi, M., and Karig, J.L. Absorption of drugs through the oral mucosa. J. Oral Ther. Pharmacol. 1965; 1:440.

Meyer, J., Squier, C.A., and Gerson, S.J. The structure and function of oral mucosa. Oxford, U.K.: Pergamon Press, 1984.

Rubright, S.C., Walker, J.A., Karlsson, U.L., and Diehl, D.L. Oral slough caused by dentifrice detergents and aggravated by drugs with antisialic activity. J. Am. Dent. Assoc., 1978; 97:215.

Schroeder, H.E., and Listgarten, M.A. Structure of the developing epithelial attachment of human teeth, vol. 2, ed. 2. New York: S. Karger, 1977.

Strachan, D.S. Histology of oral mucosa. In: Avery, J.K., Oral development and histology. Toronto: B.C. Decker, 1987.

15

Salivary Glands and Tonsils

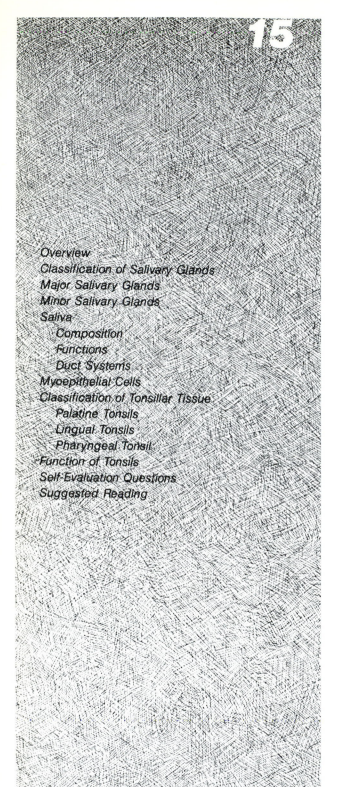

■ Overview

This chapter discusses the structure and function of the salivary glands and tonsils. Despite different structure and function, both are soft tissues contributing significantly to oral health. Saliva is a balanced secretion resulting from both (1) the composition of the secretion and (2) the location of the salivary gland secretions into the oral cavity. There are two cells types: serous, which is a high-protein low-carbohydrate, and mucous, which is a low-protein high-carbohydrate. Glands of the lips, cheeks and anterior floor of the mouth produce a watery mixture of the serous and mucous secretion, while the glands of the posterior palate, pharynx, and tongue contribute a viscous mucous solution that protects the membranes in those regions. The major salivary glands contribute 85 to 90 percent of the saliva into the more anterior area of the mouth. In addition to the protein-carbohydrate, the parotid, which is the largest gland, also secretes the enzyme amylase that aids in the digestion of carbohydrates. Therefore, the buffering ability of saliva is due to the ionic secretions by the salivary glands, which is collected and modified through an elaborate secretory duct system.

Tonsils, like the salivary glands, have locations that maximally effect and protect the oral environment. These lymph-node–like organs are positioned in the oropharynx at the entrance to the alimentary canal, where they produce lymphocytes, and along with the assistance of macrophages, protect against microbes, foreign cells, and cancer cells. Lymphocytes can recognize foreign cells and respond to them by either becoming T cells, which destroy them directly or by forming B cells, which transform into plasma cells that secrete antibodies to eliminate the foreign cells.

■ Classification of Salivary Glands

Salivary glands are classified as either major or minor depending on their size and the amount of their secretion. The **major glands** carry their secretion some distance to the oral cavity by means of a main duct. The smaller **minor glands** empty their products directly into the mouth by means of short ducts. Both are composed, however, of the same cell types, either **serous** or **mucous** or a combination of the two called **serous demilunes** (Figure 15.1). Some glands consists of pure or nearly pure serous cells, whereas others are pure mucous or a combination of serous and mucous cells.

The functional unit of the salivary gland tissue is the **alveolus** or **acinus.** An acinus is a cluster of pyramid-shaped cells, either mucous, serous, or a combination of the two, that secrete into a terminal collecting duct (Figure 15.1). This collecting duct is termed the **secretory end piece** or intercalated duct. Both the large and small glands are composed of many acini, though the larger glands contain more acini or units arranged in lobules and lobes (Figure 15.2). Each cell type provides a different type of secretion. Serous cells secrete mostly protein and small amounts of carbohydrate. This secretion also contains **zymogen granules,** precursors of the enzyme **amylase,** which functions in the breakdown of carbohydrates. Serous cell secretion has a watery consistency. Mucous cells are high in carbohydrate and low in protein and discharge a viscous product called **mucin** (Figure 15.3). When mucin mixes with watery oral fluids, it becomes mucous, causing the saliva to be thick and viscous.

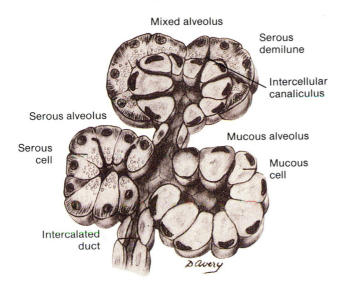

Figure 15.1 *The salivary acinar cells. The serous, mixed, and mucous alveoli are compared. Observe the cell size, shape, and position relative to the collecting tubules (intercalated duct).*

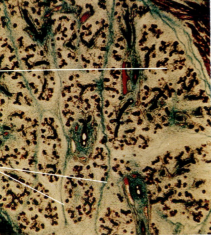

Figure 15.2 *Histology of a developing salivary gland at a stage at which the lobules can be seen outlined with connective tissue fibers (septa).*

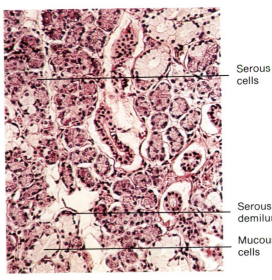

Figure 15.3 *Histologic features of the submandibular gland. Serous cells are at the upper left and mucous cells at the lower left. A few mucous cells are capped with serous cells (serous demilunes).*

Both types of acinar cells are pyramid-shaped. The nucleus of the serous cell is oval to round, and that of the mucous cell is oval to spindle-shaped (see Figure 15.1). In each of these cell types, the nuclei appear in the basal part of the cell. The cytoplasm of the serous cell stains deeply since it is filled with albumin, whereas the mucous cell appears light and foamy because of the presence of carbohydrate in mucin (Figures 15.3 and 15.4).

Ultrastructurally, the serous cell is filled with secretory granules in the apical region, rough endoplasmic reticulum, Golgi's apparatus, mitochondria, and an oval nucleus (Figure 15.5). The mucous cells contain larger droplets of mucin apically and a prominent Golgi's apparatus and rough endoplasmic reticulum around the flattened nucleus (Figure 15.6). A third cell type consists of serous cells located along the duct terminus covered with a layer of mucous cells (see Figure 15.1). The mucous secretion passes to the duct between the serous cells. This cell arrangement, called **serous demilunes,** can be seen in Figures 15.1 to 15.4).

Salivary glands are termed **merocrine glands** since the basic mode for their product's excretion is through membrane vesicles passing to the cells' apex. These vesicles fuse with the cell plasma membrane and are then exteriorized (Figure 15.6).

■ *Clinical Comment*

The serous and mucous cells of the major glands secrete 85 to 90 percent of saliva. The combined secretions produce the viscosity as well as the important buffering actions of saliva. These properties are due in part to the action of protein, carbohydrate, bicarbonate, and phosphate that is contributed by the secretory ducts of the glands.

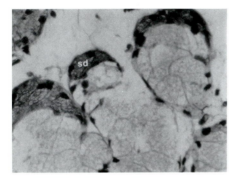

Figure 15.4 *Histology of a serous demilune (sd) cap on mucous cells in a mixed acinus of the submandibular gland.*

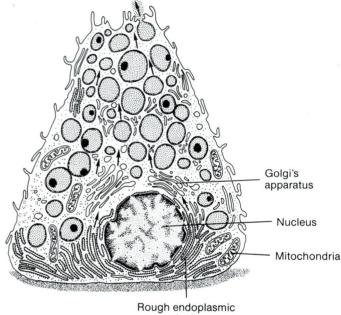
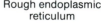

Figure 15.5 *Ultrastructure of a serous cell on the right with vesicles developing and migrating to the cell apex above. Note the round nucleus, Golgi's apparatus, and rough endoplasmic reticulum characteristic of a protein-secreting cell. (The inset shows vesicles arising from Golgi's zone.)*

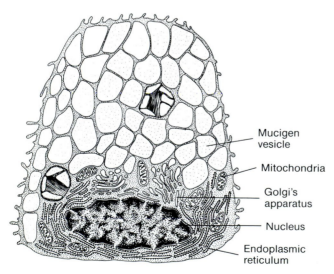

Figure 15.6 *A mucous cell. Compare the shape of this cell to that of the serous cell. Note the shape of the nucleus, the adjacent Golgi's apparatus, the rough endoplasmic reticulum, and the mucous accumulation (mucigen vesicle) in the cell.*

Major Salivary Glands

The major salivary glands are present as three bilaterally located pairs. The **parotid** glands are located on the sides of the face in front of the ears. The second pair, **submandibular,** are found inside the angle of the mandible, and the third pair, **sublingual,** are situated on either side of the midline beneath the mucosa of the anterior floor of the mouth (Figure 15.7).

Each major gland secretes a different product. The parotid produces a nearly pure serous secretion, the submandibular a mixed serous and mucous secretion, and the sublingual nearly pure mucus.

The parotids are the largest glands, although they contribute only 25 percent of the total saliva. The submandibular glands are intermediate in size, but they produce 60 percent of the saliva. The sublingual glands are the smallest, contributing only about 5 percent of the total saliva. The **minor glands,** on the other hand, contribute 5 to 10 percent of the volume of saliva.

The salivary glands are organized like grapes on a vine (Figure 15.8). The acini are the grapes, and they are arranged in groups or **lobules** invested in connective tissue. These groups of lobules form larger **lobes.** In turn, the lobes are surrounded by connective tissue containing the ducts that drain the glands as well as the blood vessels that supply the glands (Figure 15.8).

The two ducts draining the parotid glands extend anteriorly across the masseter muscles and then bend toward the mouth, opening adjacent to the crowns of the maxillary molar teeth (See Figure 15.7). The ducts of the submandibular and sublingual glands have a common opening in the anterior floor of the mouth at the sublingual papilla on either side of the frenulum and at the tongue's tip (see Figure 15.7).

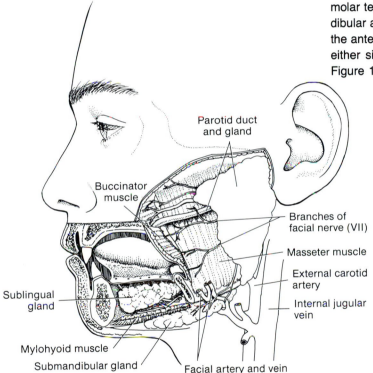

Figure 15.7 *The location of the major glands— the parotid, submandibular, and sublingual—and the relationship of the facial nerves and blood vessels to the parotid gland.*

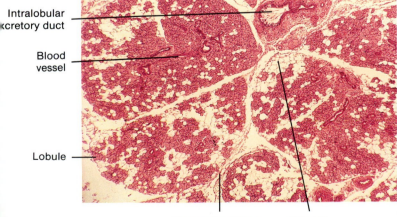

Figure 15.8 *This micrograph demonstrates the lobular nature of the parotid gland. Blood vessels can be seen within a lobule. The light lines that surround each lobule are the connective tissue fibers that support the lobules. The parotid gland contains many adipose cells (light-stained cells).*

Minor Salivary Glands

The minor salivary glands are classified as serous, mucous, or mixed types. These glands are located throughout the oral cavity and are named for their location. The glands of the cheeks and lips are termed the **buccal** and **labial glands.** They contain a combination of serous and mucous secretions and are known as **mixed glands.** The glands of both the posterior hard palate and soft palate are called **palatine glands,** and those of the tonsillar folds are the **glossopalatine glands.** These glands are referred to as **pure mucous glands.** The tongue contains **lingual glands,** which are mixed glands at the tongue's tip. Serous glands are located at the junction of the tongue's body and base where the watery secretion washes out the taste buds of the circumvallate papilla. The tongue also has mucous glands in the posterior region under the lingual tonsillar tissue. These minor glands are all shown in Figure 15.9. Each minor gland is small, consisting of a cluster of acini, and each is drained by short ducts.

■ Clinical Comment

The location of the various minor glands in the oral cavity is important to oral functions. In the palate, where keratinized epithelium is present, mucous glands provide adequate lubrication to this epithelium. The lips and cheeks have similar mixed glands that assist in swallowing and speech. The minor glands are supported by contributions from the six major glands.

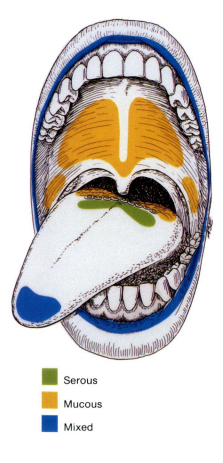

Serous

Mucous

Mixed

Figure 15.9 *The location of the minor salivary glands in the oral cavity. The serous glands are seen in the midtongue, the mucous glands in the palate, and the mixed glands in the lips, cheeks, and tongue tip.*

■ *Saliva*

Composition

All of the major and minor salivary glands contribute to the composition of saliva. This composition varies according to the rate of secretion, which is low during sleep and high (1 mil per minute ±) during stimulation. Secretion is controlled by the salivary center in the brain, and flow is generated by taste (gustatory). Masticatory function is controlled through receptors in the periodontium and muscles of mastication. Oral and pharyngeal pain and irritation can also induce stimulation.

Saliva has fewer proteins and ions than blood. Saliva contains potassium, sodium chloride, calcium, magnesium, phosphorus and bicarbonate, urea and traces of ammonia, uric acid, glucose, and lipids. The major salivary protein is amylase, which is present in the parotid gland and to a much lesser extent (20 percent) in the submandibular gland. There is none in the sublingual or minor glands. Saliva also contains the proteins lysozyme and albumin. The viscous nature of saliva is due to the presence of salivary mucin, which is a mixture of glycoproteins. Saliva contains epithelial cells shed by the oral epithelium as well as leukocytes from the gingival crevices and lymphocytes from the tonsils. The latter two are known as **salivary corpuscles.**

■ *Clinical Comment*

Saliva is important in mastication, swallowing, and speech. In addition, saliva contains amylase, an important enzyme that functions in the breakdown of carbohydrates and initiates digestive action in the oral cavity.

Functions

The three pints of saliva secreted each day serve several important functions: (1) to wash the surfaces of the teeth and reduce the possibility of acid etching leading to dental caries, (2) to keep the oral tissues moist and protect against irritants and desiccation, (3) to aid in mastication and swallowing of food, (4) to provide antibacterial action, (5) to assist in the formation of a pellicle, which is a protective membrane on the tooth's surface, and (6) to provide protection in its acid neutralizing and buffering actions, which prevent dissolution of enamel. The presence of calcium and phosphate ions in saliva increases enamel surface hardness of newly erupted teeth and may assist in enamel remineralization. Through the action of amylase, starches are broken down into more easily digestible carbohydrates. Saliva also enhances taste by breaking down food molecules into a solution that is then brought into contact with the taste buds.

Saliva has numerous proteins that have antimicrobial properties. These include lysozymes, lactoperoxidase, and lactoferrin. Additionally, saliva has antibodies or immunoglobulin such as IgA. Saliva also contains an **epidermal growth factor,** which may assist in the healing of injured oral mucosa.

During most of the day and night, salivary flow is minimal. Secretion depends on gustatory and masticatory stimulation. Both taste and smell perform a major role in determining salivary flow, as do the nerve endings in the periodontal ligament and the muscles of mastication.

■ *Clinical Comment*

The action of saliva provides an important protective function on the tooth's surface and the oral epithelium, where acids contribute to changing conditions. Saliva also contains calcium and phosphate, which may aid in the remineralization of the enamel surface and reverse the action of dental caries.

■ Duct Systems

Ducts of the smallest diameter are located in direct contact with the acini. Later, they become largest where they enter the oral cavity. The ducts of the major glands are long, and the various types of ducts in these glands are not difficult to visualize microscopically.

The ducts consist of a **secretory portion,** which lies among the acinar cells, and an **excretory portion,** which lies in the connective tissue septa between the lobules and lobes of the gland (Figure 15.10). The difference between the secretory and excretory ducts is that substances enter and leave the cells of the secretory portion by exchanging ions with the adjacent blood vessels. However, the excretory portion is simply a saliva-conducting tube. Although acinar cells drain directly into the **intercalated ducts,** which are low cuboidal cells (Figure 15.11), these secretory cells have metabolic functions and contain mitochondria, rough endoplasmic reticulum, and secretory granules. They are always located adjacent to the secretory end piece.

The next cell along the duct, the **striated duct,** is slightly taller and columnar in shape (see Figure 15.10). These cells have striations due to enfolding of the basal cell membrane, which increases their surface area (Figure 15.11). Striated duct cells readily exchange ions with the close-lying blood vessels. Sodium reabsorption and potassium secretion occur in these cells and cause changes in the composition of the saliva.

Both intercalated and striated ducts are part of the **intralobular duct system,** which is inside the lobules. In contrast, the remaining **interlobular excretory ducts** are located in the connective tissue septa between lobules and lobes of the gland (see Figures 15.8 and 15.10). As the ducts enlarge, their walls contain larger cells, such as stratified columnar cells. Near its orifice, the duct then becomes lined with stratified squamous epithelium, which is continuous with the oral epithelium. **Stensen's duct** drains the parotid gland, and **Wharton's duct** drains the submandibular gland.

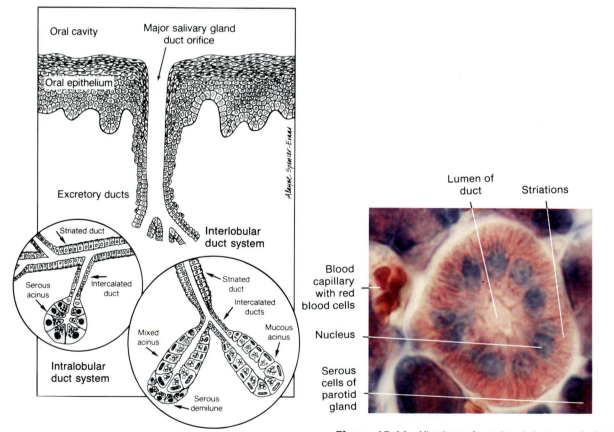

Figure 15.10 *The duct system of the salivary glands. Below are the intralobular ducts—that is, the intercalated and striated secretory ducts located within the lobule—and above are the larger interlobular, multicelled excretory ducts located outside the lobules and lobes.*

Figure 15.11 *Histology of a striated duct seen in the center of the field surrounded by parotid acinar cells. In the duct cell, note the centrally located nucleus with basal striations on the periphery of each cell. This enfolding of the cell surface provides a larger cell area to exchange nutrients with the adjacent vascular supply.*

■ *Myoepithelial Cells*

Myoepithelial cells originate from the oral epithelium at the time the epithelial cells of the salivary gland grow into the mesenchyme. They remain on the outside of the secretory end pieces to function as muscle cells in contracting or squeezing the acinus to facilitate secretion. Therefore, the term **myoepithelial cells** is used because these cells have an epithelial origin and a muscle function. These cells have long processes that wrap around the acinar and the intercalated duct cells (Figures 15.12 and 15.13). Their large nucleus and cytoplasm containing microfilaments enable them to act as smooth muscle cells.

■ *Clinical Comment*

Drugs such as tranquilizers, barbiturates, and antihistamines decrease salivary flow. In some older patients who may already have deficient salivary flow, this could be a cause of dry mouth (xerostomia).

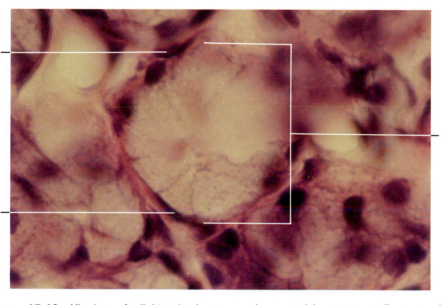

Myoepithelial cell

Myoepithelial cell

Mucous acinus

Figure 15.12 *Histology of a light-stained mucous acinus containing mucous cells surrounded by a myoepithelial cell.*

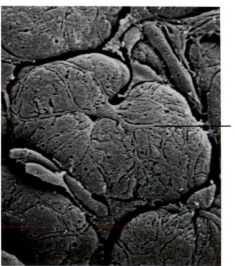

Myoepithelial cell processes

Figure 15.13 *A scanning electron micrograph of a myoepithelial cell illustrating the cell and its cytoplasmic processes wrapping around the acinus of the submandibular gland acinus.*

■ *Classification of Tonsillar Tissue*

Tonsillar tissue surrounds the oropharynx in a ring called **Waldeyer's ring.** In the oropharyngeal midline is the single **pharyngeal** tonsil or adenoid; adjacent to the posterior molars are the bilateral **palatine** tonsils; and in the floor of the mouth are the bilateral **lingual** tonsils (Figure 15.14). Tonsils are part of the lymphatic system, which also includes lymph nodes, thymus, spleen, and diffuse lymphatic tissue. Each tonsil is composed of lymphocyte masses arranged as either diffuse masses of lymphatic tissue or nodules. The lymphatic nodules in turn may have **germinal centers,** which are active sites of lymphocyte formation. These centers are common in the lingual and palatine tonsils. The tonsils are covered with epithelium. In the pharyngeal tonsil, it is respiratory epithelium, as it is in the nasopharynx, and in the orally located palatine and lingual tonsils, it is stratified squamous epithelium. This epithelial covering lines the grooves or clefts of each gland. Tonsils, unlike lymph nodes, have efferent lymphatic vessels draining them, but no afferent lymphatic vessels that lead to the tonsils. The tonsils are each supported by connective tissue and have associated glands underlying them.

Palatine Tonsils

The palatine tonsils are large in children and best recognized when they have become infected and bulge into the oropharynx, causing difficulty in swallowing. When these tonsils are infected and swollen, they appear red with streaks of white purulent material on their surface (Figure 15.15). They become infected largely as a result of their structure. Because palatine tonsils have deep, branching crypts in which oral bacteria may become lodged, these crypts may become plugged with lymphocytic discharge and desquamated epithelial cells. Beneath the palatine tonsils are seromucous glands, which could help flush out these crypts. Their ducts, however, open not into the tonsillar crypts but onto the surface of the glands. This lack of flushing action in the crypts may account for the accumulation of foreign debris and bacteria that cause tissue inflammation.

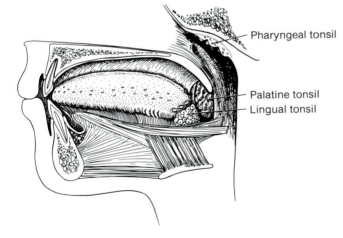

Figure 15.14 *Location of the three tonsillar groups. The palatine tonsil in the lateral wall of the oropharynx, the lingual in the midline floor of the mouth, and the pharyngeal in the midline posterior pharyngeal wall.*

Figure 15.15 *Oral view of the palatine tonsils (arrows). These tonsils are inflamed and swollen and project into the oropharyngeal cavity.*

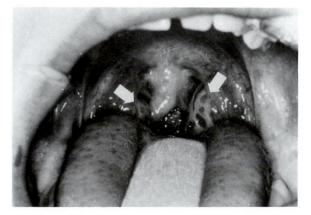

Structurally, these are the largest tonsils of the three types and are divided into lobules by the crypts. Each lobule contains numerous lymphatic nodules, which contain **germinal centers** (Figure 15.16). Septa of connective tissue support the nodules of lymphatic tissue and invest the gland in a capsule.

Lingual Tonsils

Lingual tonsils are located in the midline on the posterior third surface of the tongue (see Figure 15.14). The tonsillar mass is bilateral since it is divided in the midline reflecting the origin of the bilateral tongue. Lingual tonsils have wide-mouthed crypts that are not branching and rows of lymphatic nodules supported by connective tissue septa that are present in each lobule of the gland (Figure 15.17). These tonsils also have a connective tissue capsule investing them. The capsule is covered with nonkeratinized stratified squamous epithelium. Underlying these tonsils between the mucous glands are skeletal muscles and adipose tissue of the tongue. These mucous glands, with their ducts opening into the crypts, function in a cleansing action. Also, because these tonsils are located in the posterior floor of the mouth, the washing action of saliva provides effective cleansing. Therefore, this tonsillar mass is rarely inflamed.

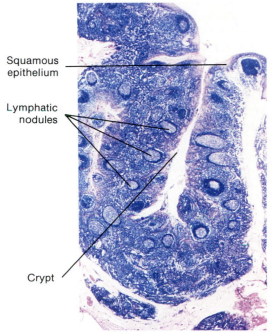

Figure 15.16 *Histology of the palatine tonsil. Observe the overlying squamous epithelium, the deep branching crypts, and the organized lymphatic nodules.*

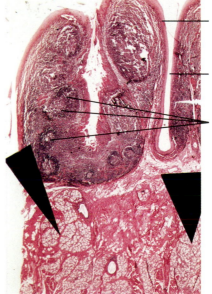

Figure 15.17 *Histology of the posterior tongue tonsil (lingual tonsil). Note the investing squamous epithelium, the short crypts, and the lymphatic nodules. Arrows denote underlying mucous glands.*

Pharyngeal Tonsil

The pharyngeal tonsil, or **adenoid,** is located in the posterior wall of the superior portion of the nasopharynx. It is subject to infection in childhood. The pharyngeal tonsil may grow laterally from its midline location to surround the opening of the auditory tube. Tonsillar tissue in this location is called the **tubal tonsil** and can be a source of infection to the eustachian tube. The pharyngeal tonsil is unlike the other tonsils in that it is an aggregation of lymphocytes that does not have crypts but has occasional folds that appear as clefts in the mucosa (Figure 15.18). This tonsil is variable in structure since only occasionally are there lymphoid nodules, which are usually only a surface accumulation of diffuse lymphoid tissue. The covering epithelium is pseudostratified columnar with occasional patches of stratified squamous. Again, this is variable since this epithelium transforms in either direction as respiratory or stratified squamous epithelium. Underlying this tonsil are mixed glands that drain on the surface of the epithelium overlying the gland tissue.

■ *Function of Tonsils*

The most notable function of tonsils is the production of lymphocytes that protect the body from foreign microorganisms inhaled or swallowed. Allergens may be sensed by these cells, which then start the complex process of coding for antibody production. Because of their ability to retain this information, lymphocytes have been called **memory cells.** Some lymphocytes transform into **T cells** and engulf the bacteria or discharge substances to destroy them. Other lymphocytes may become **B cells,** which differentiate into plasma cells. Plasma cells secrete antibodies that destroy antigens. Plasma cells along with lymphocytes are found in chronic infections such as periodontal disease, which involves the gingiva. Plasma cells found in the area of the salivary acinar cells produce IgA, which joins with the end piece of the intercellular area to form secretory IgA. Some foreign substances are taken up into the crypts of the glands into the gland proper, where they are then destroyed.

■ *Clinical Comment*

Tonsils are ideally positioned around the entrance to the alimentary canal to aid in protecting the body from invasion of microorganisms. They are important in the antibacterial action of the B and T lymphocytes and in the action of the plasma cells in the formation of secretory IgA, which neutralizes viruses and can be an antibody to food antigens.

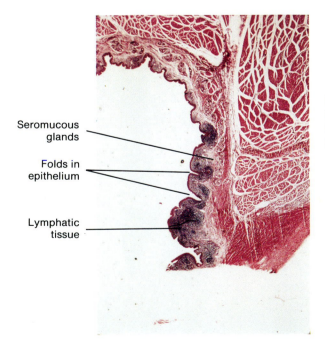

Seromucous glands

Folds in epithelium

Lymphatic tissue

Figure 15.18 *Histologic appearance of the pharyngeal tonsil with folds in epithelium rather than crypts in the tissue, diffuse lymphatic tissue rather than nodules, and seromucous glands underlying the tonsillar tissue.*

■ Self-Evaluation Questions

1. What are the location and function of myoepithelial cells?
2. Describe the two secretory ducts cells and their functions.
3. What is the contribution of the major and minor salivary glands to the total volume of saliva?
4. Compare the appearance and function of serous and mucous cells.
5. Where are most serous demilune cells found?
6. What is the origin of secretory IgA?
7. Delineate the location of the various types of minor salivary glands.
8. Describe the gland type underlying each tonsil.
9. How does gland structure relate to the causes of tonsillitis?
10. What is the function of B and T cells of the tonsils?

■ Acknowledgments

Figure 15.13 is a scanning electron micrograph study of myoepithelial cells kindly provided by Dr. T. Nagato.

Dr. D.S. Strachan contributed to Chapter 17, Nasal Cavity, Paranasal Sinuses, and Dr. R.M. Klein to Chapter 25, Development, Structure, and Function of Salivary Glands, in Avery, J.K., ed., *Oral Development and Histology,* Toronto: B.C. Decker, 1988. Some of the comments and figures used in this chapter were obtained from these sources with appreciation.

■ Suggested Reading

Drummond, J.R., and Chishiolm, D.M. A quantitative and qualitative study of the aging human labial salivary glands. Arch. Oral Biol., 1984; 29:151.

Kim, S.K., Nasjleti, C.E., and Han, S.S. The secretion process in mucous and serous secreting cells of the rat's sublingual gland. J. Ultrastruct. Res., 1972; 38:371.

Mason, D.K., and Chisholm, D.M. Salivary glands in health and disease. Philadelphia: W.B. Saunders, 1955.

Nagato, T., Yoshida HG., Yoshida A., Uehara Y. A scanning electron microscope study of the myoepithelial cells in exocrine glands. Cell Tissue Res., 1980; 209:1.

Tandler, B. Microstructure of salivary glands. In: Rowe, N.H., ed. Salivary glands and their secretion, Proceedings of a Symposium. Ann Arbor, Mich.: University of Michigan Press, 1972.

Young, J.A., and Van Lennep, E.W. The morphology of salivary glands. New York: Academic Press, 1978.

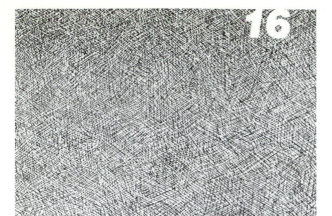

16

Pellicle, Plaque, and Calculus

■ Overview

This chapter describes substances that form on the surface of teeth and explains how they develop. The primary cuticle is of cellular origin and is formed before tooth eruption. All other products originate from saliva. The primary cuticle forms the zone of junctional epithelium; the remaining epithelium is lost soon after the teeth erupt into contact. Saliva contains salivary proteins and glycoproteins that attach to enamel or exposed cementum or dentin. Saliva then deposits a thin protein coat or membrane called a pellicle on the surface of the teeth. The pellicle, although protective to the teeth, allows plaque to form on the surface of the teeth. This plaque is composed of bacteria and salivary proteins that will become a dense layer that gradually accumulates on the tooth's surface if not removed. The bacteria in plaque may produce an acid that can cause etching and some disintegration of the enamel surface. This leads to the initiation of dental caries. Dental caries therefore develop in areas where brushing or washing of the tooth's surface does not occur. In other instances, plaque may not produce acid but may become mineralized into calculus. Calculus forms by mineralization of the remaining plaque bacteria into a hydroxyapatite deposit on enamel and exposed cementum surfaces. Continuous acquisition of calculus forms a thick deposit that should be removed, because the potential for inflammation or infection of gingival tissue could cause destructive periodontal disease.

■ *Cuticle*

The **primary** or **developmental cuticle** is deposited on the enamel's surface by the ameloblasts as their last function, shortly before the tooth crown erupts into the oral cavity. At this time, the formed enamel has reached a thickness of 2 to 2.5 mm over the cusps and is fully mineralized. In their final action, the ameloblasts secrete a thin, structureless protein membrane on the tooth's surface. On the outer surface of this cuticle is the remainder of the enamel organ cells, termed the **reduced enamel epithelium.** This cellular membrane on the tooth's surface includes the ameloblasts and other remnants of the enamel organ. Ameloblasts form the primary cuticle. The reduced enamel epithelium is lost during eruption of the teeth in the oral cavity (Figure 16.1). Only the developmental cuticle remains on the surface of the tooth as it erupts into occlusal function. However, this cuticle is not present long on the enamel, since abrasion by contact of the opposing teeth causes it to wear away. Then, only that part covering the enamel in the gingival crevice remains (Figure 16.2). This membrane serves as an attachment of the gingival junctional epithelial cells to the tooth. The sulcular epithelium is continually forming protein attachment, which renews the tooth's attachment throughout its life. Cuticular protein attachment, which initiates attachment of the junctional epithelium to the enamel, is the most important function of the primary cuticle since the rest is lost.

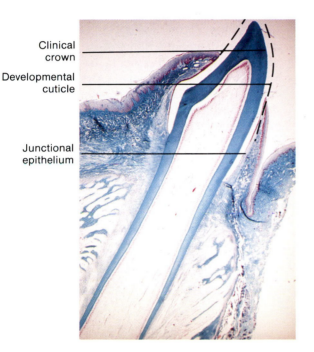

Clinical crown

Developmental cuticle

Junctional epithelium

Figure 16.1 *The crown's clinical appearance at the time the enamel is covered with the developmental cuticle.*

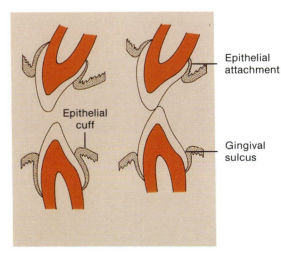

Epithelial attachment

Epithelial cuff

Gingival sulcus

Figure 16.2 *Diagram of attainment of functional occlusion illustrating the area of the gingiva's and epithelial attachment's ultimate position during tooth eruption.*

■ Acquired Pellicle

When the tooth's surface is cleansed, salivary proteins and glycoproteins, with their strong attraction for the enamel surface, are quickly deposited. The resulting layer forms a thin, structureless membrane about 0.5 to 1.0 µm thick, which is in contrast to the previously formed cuticular layer. This membrane is termed the **pellicle** or **acquired pellicle** (Figure 16.3).

Although the pellicle is bacteria free when formed, bacteria rapidly attach to its surface. The pellicle covers the entire free surface of the enamel and may penetrate any convenient defect in the tooth's surface, such as a crack, a pit, or an overhanging restoration (Figure 16.4).

Normally, the surface layers of enamel rods are straight and at right angles to the tooth surface. The zone is about 30 µm thick, with the long axis of the apatite crystals oriented nearly perpendicular to the enamel surface (Figures 16.4A and B). This area is termed the **prismless zone** of the enamel. The acquired pellicle overlying this zone has a fine, granular appearance and is approximately 500 Å thick when viewed in ultrastructure (Figure 16.4A and B).

If the pellicle is lost as a result of an oral prophylaxis, it forms again in a few minutes. Although the acquired pellicle is considered protective to the enamel surface, it does provide an attachment site for bacteria that form the plaque.

■ Clinical Comment

The bathing of the tooth's surface with saliva causes formation of a thin organic membrane, the pellicle, which in part protects the tooth's surface from the action of oral bacteria. Oral bacteria lodge anywhere there is a crevice or other defect and can attach to and penetrate the pellicle, causing enamel dissolution by acid production.

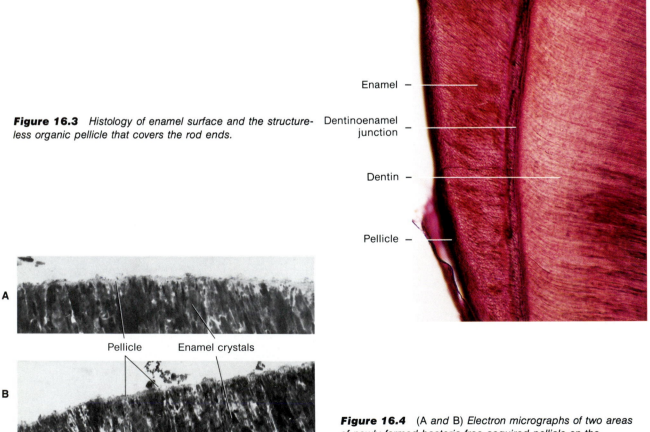

Figure 16.3 *Histology of enamel surface and the structureless organic pellicle that covers the rod ends.*

Enamel –
Dentinoenamel junction –
Dentin –
Pellicle –

Pellicle   Enamel crystals

Figure 16.4 *(A and B) Electron micrographs of two areas of newly formed bacteria-free acquired pellicle on the enamel's surface (prismless zone).*

■ *Plaque*

The central fissure of a molar, premolar, or cervical margin of any tooth is the site for accumulation and colonization of oral organisms (Figure 16.5). In addition to bacteria that attach to the pellicle, lymphocytes, leukocytes, desquamated epithelial cells, and clumps of mucin may lodge in any of these sites (Figures 16.6 and 16.7). Organisms attach to the pellicle and take advantage of debris.

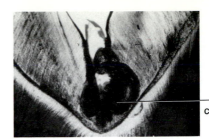

Plaque in central fissure

Figure 16.5 *Incipient carious lesion in the central fissure of the enamel in a human molar. Plaque has accumulated in this area.*

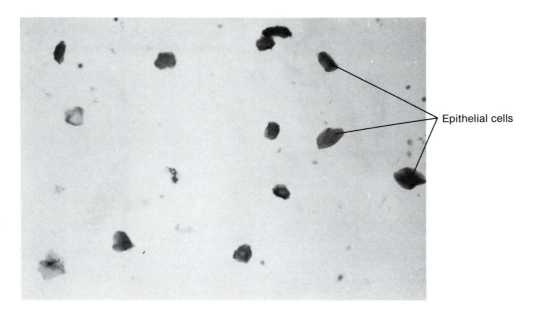

Epithelial cells

Figure 16.6 *A salivary smear viewed microscopically and showing the presence of desquamated epithelial cells.*

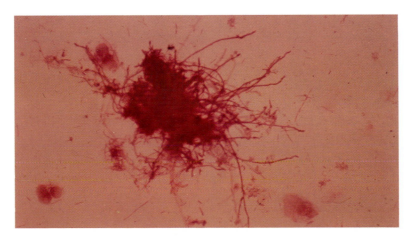

Figure 16.7 *Clumps of mucin from saliva that may adhere to crevices or imperfections in the enamel's surface.*

In the event of gingival or tonsillar inflammation, the number of lymphocytes and leukocytes increases (Figure 16.8). If a microscopic analysis of the saliva sample reveals many lymphocytes, tonsillitis is indicated. However, an increase in leukocytes in saliva is indicative of gingival inflammation. These cells are called **salivary corpuscles** (Figure 16.9). At first, there are a few bacteria on the pellicle that rapidly grow into a thick **plaque** with a variety of microorganisms. The cocci of the initial plaque quickly change in composition to include rods and filamentous organisms. These appear after only a few days, as shown in Figure 16.10. The composition of plaque depends also on the extent of gingival disease and whether the location of plaque is supragingival or subgingival. The initial carious lesions affect the prismless zone of enamel, since plaque bacteria cause dissolution of these surface crystals. A breakdown of enamel crystals is seen clinically as a brown spot on the tooth surface and as a loss of enamel rod structure microscopically, as seen in Figure 16.11. The enamel pellicle may overlie the area of an early lesion on the tooth's surface and be covered by plaque bacteria. Such a lesion may become filled with organic debris and bacteria (Figure 16.12). Note how the crystals appear to dissolve in one area and be intact in an adjacent area of enamel.

Plaque can best be seen when a **disclosing solution** is used (0.2 % basic fuchsin or erythrosin, red #3 dye) to determine if all plaque has been removed. The advantage of using red #3 dye is that it does not permanently discolor composite-type restorations or clothing. Following use of this agent and rinsing, the staining reveals any remaining plaque deposits, as observed in Figure 16.13. These visible deposits can be removed by further polishing.

■ *Clinical Comment*

Deposition of calculus can occur when the bacteria become calcified, forming a stonelike deposit. A disclosing agent can expose plaque bacteria to facilitate its removal, but plaque will reappear unless appropriate oral hygiene intervention is practiced. The removal of plaque is therefore important in the prevention of gingival and periodontal disease.

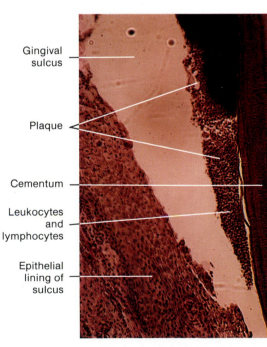

Gingival sulcus

Plaque

Cementum

Leukocytes and lymphocytes

Epithelial lining of sulcus

Figure 16.8 *The gingival sulcus viewed microscopically. Leukocytes and lymphocytes appear along the surface of the sulcus and the tooth.*

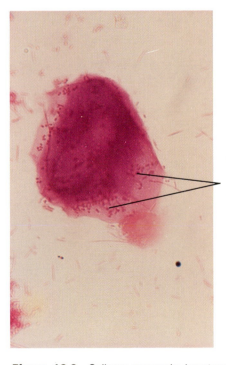

Bacteria in and on the surface of salivary corpuscle

Figure 16.9 *Salivary corpuscle: lymphocyte-containing bacteria present in the saliva.*

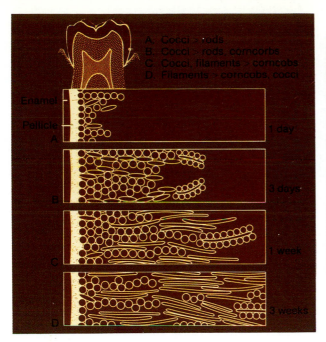

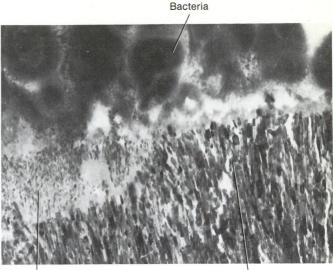

Figure 16.11 *An electron micrograph of the effects of bacteria on the enamel surface. An initial lesion is seen in the enamel surface to the left. Note the loss of enamel crystals.*

Figure 16.10 *The changes in plaque over a three-week period. In A, at one day, and in B, after three days, the cocci and a few filaments characterize the plaque. In C, after one week, the filamentous organisms appear. In D, by three weeks, the filamentous organisms predominate in the plaque.*

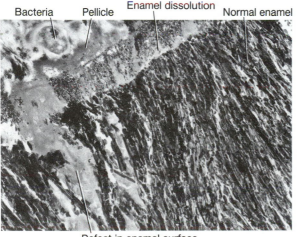

Figure 16.12 *In this electron micrograph, a penetrating carious lesion appears in the enamel (left). Initial enamel dissolution and normal enamel are seen under the pellicle and plaque (upper right).*

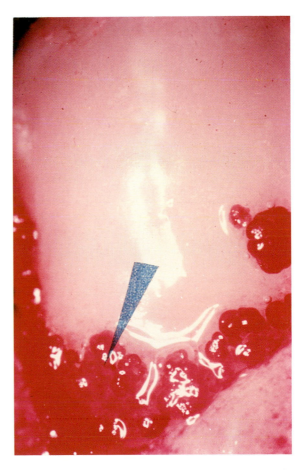

Figure 16.13 *View of the oral cavity after use of a disclosing solution. Note the presence of specific areas of stained plaque (arrowhead).*

■ *Calculus*

Calculus is a hard, stonelike concretion that forms on teeth or dental prostheses. It is primarily composed of calcium phosphate in the form of **hydroxyapatite,** which develops on the organic cell walls of bacterial plaque. Calculus formation is the reverse of enamel surface demineralization.

Calculus appears most often near the opening of the parotid excretory duct on buccal surfaces of maxillary molars and on lingual surfaces of mandibular incisors near the openings of the submandibular and sublingual gland ducts. After plaque accumulates, mineralization begins in the inner layer of the pellicle and then spreads into the overlying plaque as it thickens with further deposition of plaque protein. Note in Figure 16.14 that calcified bacteria appear as circular profiles.

Calculus deposition follows any surface irregularity of the tooth—for example, on dentin or cementum after scaling (Figure 16.15). Therefore, calculus forms in a caloospherite manner as the calcium salts derived from saliva organize within the organic skeletons of plaque bacteria. As the plaque calcifies, it loses its ability to produce an acid environment.

Calculus varies in both composition and hardness, with harder calculus containing more mineral matter. Calculus may develop above the gingival margin or within the gingival crevice. Subgingival calculus is much harder and forms more slowly than supragingival calculus. It is usually darker because it contains blood pigments.

Bacteria

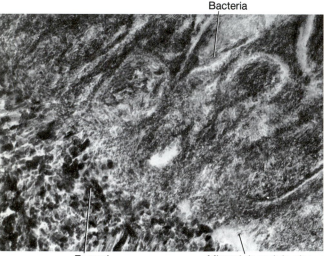

Enamel   Mineral deposit in plaque

Figure 16.14   *Calculus formation viewed by electron microscopy. Note the minute mineral crystals filling the circular bacterial ghosts on the enamel surface.*

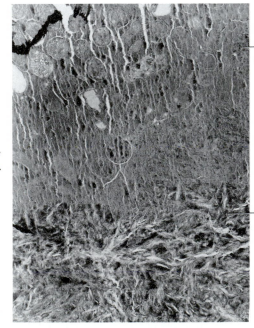

Calculus (calcified plaque)

Root dentin

Figure 16.15   *Calculus is seen on the irregular surface of dentin after root scaling. Compare the minute mineral crystals in the calculus above with the larger ones in the dentin below.*

Typical bacteria and calculus appearing in the gingival crevice are seen in Figure 16.16. Gram-positive organisms appear in the supragingival area, and gram-negative organisms are seen in the subgingival area (Figure 16.17). This is because gram-positive organisms are aerobic or living in air, whereas gram-negative organisms are anaerobic or function best without air. Bacterial action combined with the deposit results in gingival inflammation, affecting the location of the gingival attachment to the cementum rather than the cervical enamel.

■ *Clinical Comment*

Salivary calculus is damaging to the gingival tissues and should be removed by scaling. This scaling is frequently accompanied by bleeding of the gingival tissues. The gingiva heals rapidly, and the bleeding soon abates.

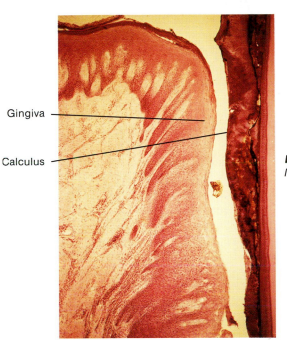

Gingiva

Calculus

Figure 16.16 *Calculus appearing in a gingival crevice relates to pocket formation.*

Figure 16.17 *This diagram compares the composition of the supragingival plaque organisms with that of the subgingival organisms. Deep in the pocket are gram-negative rods and motile spirochetes. In the area of the supragingiva and gingival margin, the rods are gram-positive.*

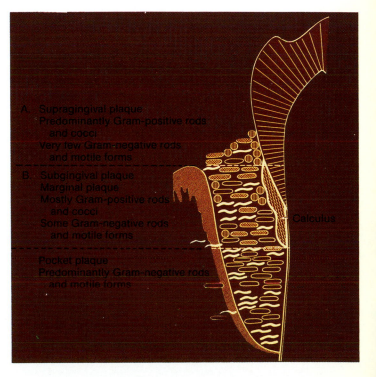

A. Supragingival plaque
   Predominantly Gram-positive rods
      and cocci
   Very few Gram-negative rods
      and motile forms

B. Subgingival plaque
   Marginal plaque
   Mostly Gram-positive rods
      and cocci
   Some Gram-negative rods
      and motile forms

   Pocket plaque
   Predominantly Gram-negative rods
      and motile forms

Calculus

■ Self-Evaluation Questions

1. Where does plaque usually form?
2. What is the composition of calculus, and how does it form?
3. Define salivary corpuscles.
4. Of what components is a pellicle composed?
5. What types of bacteria are seen supragingivally and subgingivally?
6. Define the primless zone of enamel.
7. Describe the composition of plaque bacteria and how it may change with time.
8. What is the difference between salivary and serumal calculus?
9. Discuss the purpose of using a disclosing solution.
10. How rapidly do pellicle and plaque form?

■ Acknowledgments

Figures 16.4A and B, 16.11, 16.12, and 16.14 were provided by Dr. R.F. Frank, Professor and Dean, and Dr. M. Brendel, Professor, Faculty de Chirurgie Dentaire, Strasburg, France

Figure 16.15 was provided by Dr. Knut S. Selvig, Professor and Head, Department of Dental Research, School of Dentistry, University of Bergen, Bergen, Norway.

Figures 16.10 and 16.17 were provided by Dr. Walter Loesche, Professor of Biologic and Material Sciences, The University of Michigan, School of Dentistry, Ann Arbor, Michigan.

All of the aforementioned figures were reprinted from Avery, J.K., ed. *Oral Development and History,* Toronto: B.C. Decker, 1988.

■ Suggested Reading

Listgarten, M.A. Structure of the microbial flora associated with periodontal health and disease in man. J. Periodontol. 1976; 47:1.

McHugh, W.D. Dental plaque. Edinburgh: E. & S. Livingstone, 1970.

Newman, H.N. Update on plaque and periodontal disease. J. Clin. Periodontol. 1980; 7:251.

Silverstone, L.M., Johnson, N.W., Hardie, J.M., and Williams, R.A.D. The formation, structure and microbial composition of dental plaque. In: Silverstone, L.M., Johnson, N.W., Hardie, J.M., and Williams, R.A.D. eds. Dental caries aetiology, pathology and prevention. New York: Macmillan, 1981.

Glossary

Accessory root canal. Secondary canal extending from the pulp to the surface of the root; usually found near apices of the root.

Acellular cementum. That part of the cementum covering one-third to one-half of the root of a tooth adjacent to the cementoenamel junction. It consists of collagenous fibers and ground substance.

Acinus (alveolus). A small terminal saclike dilatation particular to glands such as the salivary glands.

Acquired pellicle. An acellular organic thin skin or film deposited on the surface of teeth from salivary proteins (saliva) that bathe the surface of the teeth after eruption.

Alveolar bone. Ridge of bone; refers to tooth-bearing part of the mandible and maxilla, as it contains the tooth sockets.

Alveolar bone proper. A thin lamina of bone that lines the sockets and supports the roots of the teeth and gives attachment to principal fibers of the periodontal ligament.

Alveolar crest fibers. Those principal fibers of the periodontal ligament extending between the crest of the alveolar bone and the neck of the tooth.

Alveoli. See *Dental alveoli.*

Ameloblast. One of the differentiated cells of the inner layer of the enamel organ. There, cells give rise to the enamel of the teeth.

Amelogenesis. The process of production and development of enamel.

Amelogenin. Protein found in newly deposited enamel matrix. Amelogenins are lost during maturation of enamel.

Amylase. Enzyme that catalyzes the hydrolysis of starch into smaller water-soluble carbohydrates.

Anatomic crown. That portion of the tooth covered by enamel.

Angioblasts. Cells that give rise to blood cells and blood vessels.

Antibody. A protein produced in the body in response to invasion by a foreign agent or antigen that has a specific reaction.

Aortic arches. A series of arterial channels encircling the embryonic pharynx within the mesenchyme of the branchial arches.

Apical foramen. Opening at the apex of the tooth's root giving passage to the nerves and blood vessels.

Appositional growth (exogenous). Deposition of successive cell products laid down upon those already present.

Articular disc (of the temporomandibular joint). The fibrous disc that separates the upper and lower joint cavities.

Attached gingiva. The part of the oral mucosa that is firmly bound at the neck of the tooth and the alveolar process.

Attached pulpal stones or denticles. Mineralized tissues that are partly fused with the dentin of the coronal pulp or root canal.

B cells. Lymphocytes that have differentiated into plasma cells. Plasma cells secrete antibodies that destroy antigens.

Basal lamina. Membrane separating the epidermis and dermis that is a product of both.

Bell stage. Developmental stage of the tooth characterized by the differentiation of inner enamel epithelial cells into ameloblasts and the formation of the outline of the future crown by these cells.

Blastocyst. The postmorula stage of development; a blastula with a fluid-filled cavity.

Bone. Mineralized animal tissue consisting of an organic matrix, cells, and fibers of collagen impregnated with mineral matter, chiefly calcium phosphate and calcium carbonate. See also *Bundle bone, Cancellous bone, Compact bone, Haversian bone.*

Branchial. Barlike, resembling the gills of a fish.

Branchial arch. One of a series of mesodermal bars located between the branchial clefts. During embryonic stages, they contribute to the formation of the face, jaws, and neck. They appear in higher forms only vestigially.

Branchial arch cartilages. The cartilages found in the branchial arches of the embryo.

Bud stage. Initial stage of tooth development; the enamel organ develops from this structure. The dental papilla lies adjacent to the epithelial bud, and the dental sac encloses both.

Bundle bone. Specialized bone lining the tooth socket into which the fibers of the periodontal ligament penetrate. The radiographic term *lamina dura* is synonymous with *bundle bone.*

Calcification. See *Diffuse calcification.*

Calculus. An abnormal concretion within the body, usually formed of mineral salts and often deposited around a minute fragment of inorganic material, the nucleus. See also *Dental calculus, Serumal calculus.*

Canals. See *Haversian canals.*

Cancellous bone. Spongy or lattice-like structure composed mainly of bone tissue.

Cap stage. In tooth development, an early stage in enamel organ formation; follows the bud stage.

Cartilage. Fibrous connective tissue characterized by nonvascularity and a firm consistency. Forms most of the temporary skeleton of the embryo. See also *Hyaline cartilage.*

Cell. Smallest unit of living structure capable of independent existence.

Cell-free zone. Relatively cell-free layer of the dental pulp adjacent to odontoblasts and overlying the cell-rich zone. Composed of delicate fibrils in ground substance.

Cell-rich zone. Layer of the dental pulp situated between the pulp core and the cell-free zone, which is richly supplied with cellular elements, blood vessels, and nerves.

Cellular cementum. That part of the cementum covering the apical one-half to two-thirds of the root of a tooth. This cementum is most abundant on the root tip.

Cementicles. Calcified spherical bodies composed of cementum lying either free within the periodontal ligament, attached to the cementum, or embedded within it.

Cementoblast. A large cuboidal cell lying on the surface of the bone that is active in cementum formation.

Cementocyte. A cell found in the lacuna of cellular cementum. Numerous cytoplasmic processes extend from its free surface.

Cementoid layer. See *Intermediate cementum.*

Cementum. Bonelike connective tissue that covers the tooth from the cementoenamel junction to and surrounding the apical foramen. See also *Acellular cementum, Cellular cementum.*

Central nervous system (CNS). Composed of the brain and spinal cord.

Centriole. Either of two short cylinders appearing near the nucleus that migrate to opposite poles of the cell during cell division.

Cervical loop. Growing free border of the enamel organ. Here, the outer and inner enamel epithelial cell layers are continuous with each other.

Chromosome. A structure in the nucleus containing a thread of DNA during cell division, providing genetic information.

Circumpulpal dentin. Inner portion of the dentin located near the pulp organ of the tooth.

Clinical crown. That portion of the crown exposed and visible in the oral cavity.

CNS See *Central nervous system (CNS).*

Col. Valley-like depression in the facial lingual plane of the interdental gingiva. It conforms to the shape of the interproximal contact area.

Collagen. White fibers of the corium of the skin, tendon, and other connective tissue. The fiber is composed of fibrils bound with interfibrillar cement.

Collagen fiber. High-molecular-weight protein composed of several structural types that vary in diameter and usually are arranged in bundles.

Compact bone. Dense bone more highly calcified than cancellous (spongy) bone.

Condyle. See *Mandibular condyle.*

Coronal pulp. That pulp present in the crown of a tooth.

Cranial. Pertaining to the cranium, specifically those bones covering the brain.

Cranial base. Lower portion of the skull constituting the floor of the cranial cavity.

Crypts. Pitlike depressions or tubular recesses on a free surface.

Cuticle. See *Primary cuticle.*

Cytoplasm. Protoplasm of a cell located in the area surrounding the nucleus.

Dead tracts. Empty tubules resulting from loss of the odontoblastic processes.

Deciduous dentition. Primary teeth that function during the first eight years of life and then exfoliate, providing space for the permanent teeth.

Dehiscence. Alveolar bone loss in the coronal root.

Demilune. A crescent-shaped structure or cell. See also *Serous demilune.*

Dendrite. Component of the neuron that receives and conducts impulses to the cell body.

Dental alveoli. The alveoli or sockets in which the roots of teeth are embedded.

Dental calculus. Hard stonelike concretion formed on the teeth, on a prosthesis, or in salivary ducts. It varies in color from creamy yellow to black and is mostly composed of calcium phosphate.

Dental lamina. Horseshoe-shaped epithelial bands that traverse the upper and lower jaws and give rise to the ectodermal portions of the teeth.

Dental papilla. Part of the formative organ of the teeth that forms the dentin and the pulp.

Dental plaque. Organic deposit on the surface of teeth. Site of bacterial growth and formation of dental calculus.

Dental pulp. The soft tissue contained within the pulp chamber. Consists of connective tissue, blood vessels, nerves, and lymphatics.

Dental sac (follicle). Area of mesenchymal cells and fibers that surround the dental papilla and the enamel organ of the developing teeth. It produces the periodontal ligament, alveolar bone, and cementum.

Dentin. Yellowish body of the tooth; surrounds the pulp and underlies the enamel on the crown and the cementum on the roots of the teeth. Composed of 20 percent organic matrix, mostly collagen, and 10 percent water. The inorganic fraction (70 percent) is hydroxyapatite, with some carbonate, magnesium, and fluoride. See also *Intratubular or peritubular dentin* and *Mantle dentin.*

Dentinoenamel junction. Interface of the enamel and dentin of the crown of a tooth.

Dentinogenesis. The process of dentin formation in the development of teeth.

Dermatomes. Dorsal lateral portion of the somite of the embryo. These cells form the dermis, subcutaneous tissue, and supporting tissue of the gastrointestinal tract.

Dermis. Arises from the mesoderm underlying the epidermis. The dermis and the epidermis together form the skin.

Desmosome. Cell junction. It consists of a dense plate near the cell surface that relates to a similar structure on an adjacent cell, between which are thin layers of extracellular material.

Diaphysis. The shaft of the long bone.

Differentiation. Process by which cells acquire individual cellular characteristics from an undifferentiated state—that is, specialization.

Diffuse calcification. Irregular calcified deposits along collagen fiber bundles or blood vessels in the pulp or elsewhere. It is considered a pathologic condition.

Diphyodont. Species that develops two separate dentitions during a lifetime.

Direct innervation. Theory based on the belief that nerves may extend to the dentinoenamel junction from the pulp.

DNA (deoxyribonucleic acid). Contains the genetic information in the cell.

Drift. Movement of a tooth to a position of greater stability.

Duct. Tube with well-defined walls for passage of excretions or secretions.

Dystrophy. Any disorder arising from defective or faulty nutrition.

Ectomesenchyme. Neural crest cells, mesectoderm. Forms spinal ganglia.

Edentulous jaw. Alveolar bone without teeth.

Eleidin. A protein allied to keratin and protoplasm but more transparent than protein keratin.

Embryonic period. The second to eighth weeks of prenatal life.

Enamel. See *Gnarled enamel.*

Enamel crystals. Hydroxyapatite crystals found in enamel rods. They are formed during tooth mineralization.

Enamel lamellae. Thin leaflike spaces that extend from the enamel surface toward the dentinoenamel junction. They represent defects or organic filled spaces in the enamel.

Enamel organ. Originates from the dental lamina and consists of four distinct layers.

Enamel pearls. Enameloma, a developmental anomaly in which a small nodule of enamel is formed near the cementoenamel junction, usually at the bifurcation zone of molar teeth.

Enamel rod. One of the structural units of enamel, extending from the dentinoenamel junction to the surface of the tooth and normally having a translucent crystalline appearance.

Enamel spindles. Tubular spaces in enamel found at the dentinoenamel junction in which a terminal extension of the odontoblastic processes can be found.

Enamel tuft. Narrow ribbon-like structures whose constricted inner end arises at or near right angles to the dentinoenamel junction and extends one-third into the thickness of the enamel. Tufts consist of hypocalcified spaces that may be filled with organic substance.

Enamelin. The organic protein component of enamel.

Enameloid. A thin, structureless layer of substance deposited by the root sheath that may be a form of enamel.

Endochondral. Relating to the type of bone formation that occurs within cartilage and replaces it.

Endocrine. Refers to glands of internal secretion that release their secretory product(s) hormones directly into the blood stream rather than through a duct system.

Endometrium. The mucous membrane lining the uterus.

Endoplasmic reticulum (ER). An ultrastructural organelle consisting of membrane-bound cavities in the cytoplasm of the cell.

Epidermis. The surface nonvascular cell layer of the skin that develops from the surface ectodermal cells. It consists of five layers; from the inner to the outer layer, they are (1) basal, (2) spinous, (3) granular, (4) clear (lucidum), and (5) horny (corneum).

Epiphysis. The extremity of a long bone as opposed to the shaft (diaphysis).

Epithelial attachment. Attachment of the gingival epithelium with the tooth's surface at the dentogingival junction.

Epithelial cell rests. Remains of the epithelial root sheath that cover the roots during root development. Later they are located in the periodontal ligament near the surface of the cementum. Occasionally, they may develop into dental cysts. The cell groups are of these types: (1) resting, (2) proliferating, (3) degenerating.

Epithelial diaphragm. Formed by the root sheath at the beginning of root development. This structure is important during root formation. It narrows the width of the cervical opening of the root.

Epithelial pearls. Discrete rounded or ovoid groups of epithelial cells, frequently keratinized, found in the lamina propria.

Epithelial root sheath. Cervical loop enamel organ cells that proliferate, forming a double layer of cells (Hertwig's) that function in root formation.

Epithelium. Cellular avascular layer covering all the free surfaces of the body, internal and external, and the lining of vessels. Consists of cells and small amounts of intercellular substance. See also *Inner enamel epithelium.*

Eruption. See *Tooth eruption.*

Exfoliate. To shed or eliminate something from the surface of the body, as in the loss of teeth from the jaws.

Exocrine. Denotes glands that release their secretory product(s) into a duct system.

Exocytosis. Discharge of secretory product(s) from the cell, preserving the cell membrane through fusion of the secretory vesicles with the cell membrane.

Fenestration. The area of alveolar bone loss where an apical root penetrates the bone.

Fetal period. The embryo from the eighth prenatal week to birth.

Fibroblastoclasts. Those fibroblasts that can both form and destroy collagen fibers.

Fibroblasts. Elongated, ovoid, spindle-shaped, or flattened cells found in connective tissue.

Filiform papillae. The most numerous papillae appearing on the dorsum of the tongue. These threadlike elevations point dorsally and toward the throat.

Fontanelle. One of several membrane-covered spaces found in the incompletely ossified skull of the fetus or newborn.

Fordyce's spots. A condition characterized by minute yellowish white papules (sebaceous glands) on the oral mucosa.

Free gingiva. The portion of the gingiva that surrounds the tooth and is not directly attached to the tooth surface; the outer wall of the gingival sulcus.

Fundic bone. Bone enclosing the apex of the tooth root.

Fungiform papilla. One of numerous minute elevations on the dorsum, tip, and sides of the tongue. The papillae are mushroom-shaped, with the top being broader than the base.

Ganglion. A group of nerve cell bodies located outside the central nervous system.

Gap junctions. Specialized communicating junctions between cells with pores permeable to ions and small molecules.

Gingiva. Soft tissue surrounding the necks of erupted teeth that cover the alveolar process. The gingiva consists of fibrous connective tissue enveloped by mucous membrane. See also *Attached gingiva, Free gingiva, Interdental gingiva.*

Gingival sulcus. The shallow *V*-shaped trench around each tooth, bound by the tooth on one surface and the epithelium-lined free margin on the other.

Gland. See *Merocrine gland.*

Globular dentin. Areas of defective growth with interglobular spaces that underlie the enamel and surface of the root.

Gnarled enamel. The enamel located at the tips of the cusps, in which the rods or groups of rods are twisted, bent, and intertwined; seen ultrastructurally.

Golgi's apparatus or complex. A continuation of the endoplasmic reticulum. A cuplike structure within cells made up of saccules where carbohydrate side chains of glycoproteins form.

Granular layer of Tomes. A thin, granular-appearing layer of defective dentin located along the root surface adjacent to the cementum.

Gubernacular cord. Fibrous connective tissue band uniting the tooth sac with the alveolar mucosa. This cord is something that guides.

Hard palate. Anterior part of the palate consisting of the bony palate bound above by the nasal cavity and below by the mouth. It is covered by keratinized stratified squamous epithelium. In addition, the hard palate contains palatine vessels and nerves, adipose tissue, and mucous glands.

Haversian bone. Compact bone containing tubular channels with blood vessels, nerves, and bone cells surrounded by concentrically located lacunae. These structures are termed the haversian system.

Haversian canals. These nutrient canals are located in cortical bone and extend in the direction of the tooth's long axis.

Hemidesmosome. Half of a desmosome that forms a site of attachment between epithelial cells and the basal lamina or between epithelial cells (junctional cells) and the tooth's surface.

Hormone. Chemical substance formed in one organ or part of the body and carried by the blood stream to another part where it stimulates or depresses activity.

Howship's lacunae. Absorption lacunae. Tiny cup-shaped depressions on the resorbing front of any hard tissue, the result of resorptive activity by osteoclasts.

Hunter-Schreger bands. Alternating dark and light bands in enamel that result from absorption and reflection of light caused by differences in orientation of adjacent groups of enamel rods originating at the dentinoenamel junction and extending toward the outer enamel surface.

Hyaline cartilage. A flexible semitransparent elastic substance composed of a collagen fibrillar matrix, and chondrocytes in lacunae.

Hydrodynamic. Science of factors determining the flow of liquids. In dentistry, it refers to a theory of pain conduction through dentin resulting from odontoblastic movement contacting nerve endings.

Hydroxyapatite. An inorganic compound that constitutes bone and teeth.

IgA. A distinct class of immunoglobulins. A protein of animal origin with known antibody activity, synthesized by lymphocytes and plasma cells; found in serum, other body fluids, and tissues.

Imbrication lines. Also known as **von Ebner's lines.** Incremental lines in dentin that run at right angles to the tubules. These lines, which represent the daily growth pattern, indicate layers of dentin that are less calcified and appear darker than adjacent dentin.

Impaction. Position of a tooth in the alveolus so that it is incapable of eruption into the oral cavity.

Incisor liability. The succession of larger permanent incisors replacing primary ones. The size ratio of the two incisors of the two dentitions.

Increment. The amount by which a given quantity is increased. A measurable amount.

Incremental deposition. Deposition of material in discrete amounts rather than constant deposition. Rhythmic recurrent deposition of enamel, bone, dentin, or cementum.

Incremental line. An evident line produced through a rhythmic, recurrent deposition of successive layers upon those present.

Inner enamel epithelium. Cells that line the concavity of the enamel organ in the cap and early bell stages of tooth development and differentiate into ameloblasts.

Innervation. Presence and distribution of nerves within a part or the supply of nerves stimulating a part.

Intercellular tissue. Tissue located between or among cells of any structure.

Interdental gingiva. The soft tissue between adjacent contacting teeth in the same arch.

Interdental septa. Bony partitions that project into the alveoli between the teeth; interalveolar.

Intermediate cementum. A deposition by the epithelial root sheath cells on the root surface formed during root formation. May be termed *enameloid.*

Interstitial growth (endogenous). Growth by expansion of the matrix by cell deposits within the matrix.

Interstitial spaces. Spaces between groups or bundles of periodontal fibers.

Intramembranous. Within a membrane. Bone formation occurring within or among connective tissue fibers. It does not replace cartilage, as does endochondral bone.

Intratubular or peritubular dentin. The dentinal matrix that immediately surrounds the dentinal tubule.

Junctional epithelium. Epithelial attachment. That epithelium adhering to the tooth surface at the bottom of the gingival crevice and consisting of one or more layers of nonkeratinizing cells.

Keratinized. Having developed a horny layer of flattened epithelial cells containing keratin.

Keratinized mucosa. Stratified surface of cornified epithelial cells that lack a nucleus and whose cytoplasm is replaced by large amounts of keratohyalin protein.

Keratinocytes. Cells of the oral mucosa. These epidermal cells synthesize keratin.

Lacunae. The very small cavities in bone that are filled with bone cells. See *Howship's lacunae.*

Lamella. Thin leaf or plate, as of bone. See also *Enamel lamina.*

Lamina dura. A thin layer of hard compact bone lining the tooth sockets. Used in radiography to designate a thin radiopaque line.

Lamina propria. Layer of connective tissue underlying the epithelium of skin or a mucous membrane.

Langerhans' cells. Clear or dendritic cells found in both superficial and deep layers of the epidermis and oral epithelium.

Leeway space. The difference in the space in the arch required for the two primary molars and the successional permanent premolars replacing them. The leeway space in the maxilla is 1.3 mm and in the mandible 3.1 mm.

Lining mucosa. Nonkeratinized oral mucosa that covers the surface of the cheeks, lips, soft palate, floor of the mouth, and ventral surface of the tongue.

Lysosome. Small membrane-bound body that contains a variety of acid hydrolases, which function in breaking down substances both inside and outside the cell. It is seen by electron microscopy.

Macroglossia. Enlargement of the tongue that can be due to muscular hypertrophy.

Macrognathia. Excessive size of the jaw.

Macrophages. Any of the large mononuclear phagocytic cells found in various tissues and organs of the body. These cells are a normal constituent of the pulp and function in tissue maintenance.

Malassez's rests. Epithelial cell remnants of Hertwig's sheath in the periodontal ligament. These cell groups appear near the surface of the cementum; they may develop into dental cysts.

Mandible. Horseshoe-shaped bone forming the lower jaw and articulating the condyles, with the temporal bone on either side. The mandible is composed of the horizontal body and inclined ramus. The body includes the alveolar process, which contains the teeth.

Mandibular condyle. The rounded bony projection of the mandible that articulates with the temporal fossa of the temporal bone in the temporomandibular fossa.

Mantle dentin. The initially deposited portions of the dentin formed immediately adjacent to the enamel.

Masticatory mucosa. The mucosa that functions in mastication. It tends to be bound to bone and is therefore immovable. This mucosa covers the hard palate and the gingiva.

Maturation zone. Zone of cartilage characterized by chondrocyte enlargement.

Maxilla. Upper jaw bone; an irregularly shaped bone articulating with the nasal, lacrimal, zygomatic, palatine, ethmoid, sphenoid, and frontal bones of the face and containing teeth.

Maxillary sinus. Paired sinus cavities occupying the space beneath the floor of the orbit and above the roots of the posterior maxillary molars.

Meckel's cartilage. The initial skeletal component of the first branchial arch. It is the supporting cartilage of the mandibular arch in the embryo.

Medial nasal process. The area of the nose in the embryo. The tissue medial to the naris.

Median raphe. The line denoting union of the palatine bones in the midline of the palate. There is no submucosa under the palatal mucosa in this area.

Meiosis. Process of reduction division of chromosomes in the daughter cell, with half as many as in the parent cell.

Melanocytes. Cells responsible for synthesis of melanin that provide pigmentation to the skin.

Merkel's cells. Cells located in the basal layer of the gingival epithelium and thought to be epithelial in origin. They function as touch receptors.

Merocrine gland. The secreting cells remain intact during the formation and release of the secretory product.

Mesenchyme. Loose undifferentiated embryonic connective tissue that is a mixture of mesodermal and neural crest cells. The connective tissues of the body form from this tissue.

Mesial drift. General movement of a tooth or teeth anteriorly toward the midline of the jaw.

Mesoderm. The third primary germ layer of the embryo to differentiate. It is positioned between the ectoderm and endoderm. From mesoderm are derived connective tissues, bone, cartilage, muscle, blood and blood vessels, lymphatics, notochord, pleura, and peritoneum.

Microglossia. Smallness of the tongue.

Micrognathia. Smallness of the jaw, especially the mandible.

Microtubules. Small tubular structures found in the cytoplasm and composed of the protein tubulin. They are cylindrical and hollow.

Mitochondrion. Small spherical organelle that is a membrane-bound structure lying free in the cytoplasm and present in all cells. This structure is the principal site of energy generation in the cell.

Mixed dentition. Simultaneous possession of both primary and permanent teeth.

Morula. Mass of blastomeres resulting from the early cleavage divisions of the zygote.

MPD. Myofacial pain dysfunction.

Mucin. A glycoprotein that is the primary constituent of mucus.

Mucoceles. Retention cysts of the minor salivary gland ducts, which contain mucous secretion. They usually result from rupture of the excretory duct of a minor salivary gland, causing pooling of saliva in the tissues. The resulting vesicular elevation is a mucocele.

Mucous acinus. Minute saclike secretory portion of a mucous gland. This is the functional unit of the gland.

Mucous glands. Glands that produce viscous proteinaceous secretions, such as the sublingual gland and glands of the hard palate.

Myoblast. An embryonic cell that becomes a cell of muscle fiber.

Myoepithelial cells. Spindle-shaped contractive epithelial cells with stellate bodies and processes found in salivary and sweat glands. They are located in the terminal portion of the salivary gland acini and are believed to have contractile ability that facilitates movement of the glandular secretion into the ducts.

Myofibrils. Fine longitudinal fibrils (parallel to the long axis) found in a muscle fiber. They are composed of numerous myofilaments.

Nasal fin. A zone of epithelial contact of the medial nasal and maxillary processes during development.

Neonatal line. Accentuated incremental or hesitation line seen in bone, dentin, and enamel; probably due to changes occurring at or near birth.

Nerves. Whitish cords composed of fibers arranged in bundles (fascicles) and held together by a connective tissue sheath, the perineurium. The fascicles are surrounded by epineurium. Nerves transmit stimuli from the central nervous system to the periphery by the efferent motor system or from the periphery to the central nervous system by the afferent sensory system.

Neural crest. Ganglionic crest; a band of ectodermal cells that appear along either side of the embryonic neural tube at the time of closure.

Neuroblasts. Primitive nerve cells that develop into adult nerve cells, the neurons. They are the functional cells of the brain. spinal cord, and peripheral nerves.

Neurocranium. That part of the skull enclosing the brain, as distinguished from the bones of the face.

Neuroglia. The supporting structure of the brain and spinal cord, composed of specialized cells and their processes.

Neuron. A nerve cell; any of the conducting cells of the nervous system, consisting of a cell body, containing the nucleus and its surrounding cytoplasm, the dendrite, which carries impulses to the cell body, and the axon, which conducts impulses away from the cell body to the area of synapse.

Nonkeratinized mucosa. Lining mucosa in which the stratified squamous epithelial cells retain their nuclei and cytoplasm. Lining mucosa is found on the inner lips, cheeks, soft palate, vestibular fornix, alveolar mucosa, floor of the mouth, and undersurface of the tongue.

Nonkeratinocytes. Cells not producing keratin. Clear or dendritic cells found in oral epithelium such as pigment cells (melanocytes), Langerhans' cells, Merkel's cells, and inflammatory cells such as lymphocytes.

Nucleolus. A round vacuole-like achromatic body rich in RNA found within the nucleus of a cell.

Nucleus. A spheroid body within a cell, containing the genetic matter DNA, organelles, one or more nucleoli, chromatin, linin, and nucleoplasm. It has a thin nuclear membrane vital to protein synthesis.

Occlusion. Relation of the functional contact of the maxillary and mandibular teeth during activity of the mandible.

Odontoblast. One of a layer of columnar cells with long processes extending into the dentinal tubules and lining the peripheral pulp of a tooth. These cells function in dentin formation and vitalize this tissue.

Odontoblastic process. A cytoplasmic extension of the cell body of the odontoblasts, some of which extend from the cell possibly as far as the dentinoenamel junction or the cementoenamel junction.

Odontogenic zone. This area is located peripherally adjacent to the dentin in both the coronal and radicular pulp. It contains the formative cells of dentin known as odontoblasts.

Olfactory mucosa. Site of most receptors for the sense of smell. It occupies the superior aspect of the nasal cavity between the superior nasal conchae, roof of the nose, and upper part of the nasal septum.

Organelles. Living particles located in the cytoplasm of cells. They include mitochondria, Golgi's complex, centrosomes, lysosomes, ribosomes, centrioles, endoplasmic reticulum, microtubules, and microfilaments.

Organic matrix. Formative portion of a tooth or bone as opposed to mineralized hydroxyapatite.

Osteoblasts. Bone-forming cells derived from mesenchyme. They form the osseous matrix in which they may become enclosed to become osteocytes.

Osteoclasts. Multinucleated cells larger than osteoblasts derived from monocytes from the blood stream. Osteoclasts contain abundant acidophilic cytoplasm formed in bone marrow and function in the absorption and removal of osseous tissue.

Osteocytes. Cells of the bone located within lacunae, functioning in maintenance and vitality of bone.

Osteodentin. Dentin that appears more like bone than dentin since it contains cells.

Oxytalan fibers. Type of connective tissue fibers chemically different from collagen fibers and found in the periodontal ligament and gingiva. They appear similar to immature elastic fibers. These fibers are believed to support blood vessels and the principal fibers of the ligament.

Palatal rugae. Transverse ridges located in the mucous membrane of the anterior part of the hard palate. They extend laterally from the incisive papillae and have a core of dense connective tissue.

Palate. See *Primary palate, Secondary palate.*

Palatine tonsils. Two large oval masses of lymphoid tissue embedded in the lateral wall of the oropharynx bilaterally located between the pillars of the fauces.

Papillae. Small protuberances located on the tongue that are sensitive eminences, possessing a tactile function.

Parasympathetic nervous system. The craniosacral portion of the autonomic nervous system, its preganglionic fibers traveling with cranial nerves II, VII, IX, X, and XI and with the second to fourth sacral ventral roots. It innervates the heart; smooth muscle and glands of the head and neck; and thoracic, abdominal, and pelvic viscera.

Parenchyma. The functional elements of an organ rather than the supporting framework (stroma) of the organ.

Parotid. Serous secreting salivary gland located anterior to the ear. It is encapsulated and produces 26 percent of the secretions of the major salivary glands.

Pellicle. See *Acquired pellicle.*

Perforating fibers (Sharpey's fibers). Penetrating connective tissue fibers by which the tooth is attached to the adjacent alveolar bone. These bundles of collagen fibers penetrate both the cementum and the alveolar bone.

Perikymata. Wavelike transverse grooves and ridges believed to be manifestations of the striae of Retzius, on the surface of enamel. They appear transverse to the long axis of the crown.

Perimysium. Connective tissue demarcating a fascicle of skeletal muscle fibers.

Periodontal ligament. Connective tissue ligament that is a mode of attachment of the tooth to the alveolus and consists of collagenous fiber bundles. Between the bundles are loose connective tissue, blood vessels, and nerves.

Periodontium. Those tissues surrounding and supporting the teeth. There are two distinct sections: the gingival unit, composed of the free and attached gingivae and the alveolar mucosa, and the other section known as the attachment apparatus of the teeth, which includes the cementum, periodontal ligament, and alveolar process.

Peritubular dentin. The zone of dentin forming the wall of the dentinal tubules. This dentin has a 9 percent higher mineral content than does the remainder of the intertubular dentin.

Phagocytize. To engulf and destroy bacteria and other foreign substances, denoting the action of the phagocytic cells.

Pharyngeal tonsil. A collection of more or less closely aggregated lymphoid cells located superficially in the posterior wall of the nasopharynx, the hypertrophy of which constitutes the condition called adenoids.

Plaque. See *Dental plaque.*

Plasma cells. Cells derived from B lymphocytes, which actively synthesize and secrete immunoglobulins from an extensive rough endoplasmic reticulum. Under appropriate conditions, antigen stimulation induces proliferation and morphologic alteration in B lymphocytes to form plasma cells.

Plasma membrane or plasmalemma (cell membrane). Envelops the entire cell and provides a selective barrier that regulates transport of substances into and out of the cell.

Predentin. Band of newly formed, and as yet unmineralized, matrix of dentin located at the pulpal border of the dentin.

Pre-eruptive phase. Developmental stage preparatory to eruption of teeth and characterized by movements of the growing teeth within the alveolar process.

Primary cuticle. A thin film on the enamel surface of an unerupted tooth. It is the product of the degenerating ameloblasts.

Primary palate. That part of the palate formed from the median nasal process. The first palate to form that is anterior to the secondary palate.

Prismless enamel. Enamel having been formed without any rods or prism pattern.

Proliferative period. Time during which cells grow and increase in number by cell division.

Ptyalin. Synonymous term for *salivary amylase,* the enzyme in saliva that catalyzes the hydrolysis of starch into water-soluble carbohydrates.

Pulp bifurcation. Zone of branching of the pulp organ, as found in multirooted teeth.

Pulp organ. Soft tissue within the tooth, consisting of connective tissue, blood vessels, nerves, and lymphatics.

Pulpal blood vessels. Characteristic thin-walled blood vessels of the dental pulp.

Pulpal stones or denticles. Calcified mass of dentinlike substance located within the pulp or embedded in or attached to the dentinal wall. They appear as a function of age or trauma. These stones may be free, embedded, or attached to the dentin.

Quiescent stage. A period of inactivity.

Radiation. Transmission of rays: light rays, short radio-waves, ultraviolet rays, or x-rays.

Radicular pulp. The pulp occupying the root canals that extend from the cervical coronal region to the apex of the root.

Ramus. General term to designate a smaller structure given off a larger one or one into which a larger structure divides.

Ramus of mandible. Quadrilateral process projecting posteriorly and superiorly from the body of the mandible.

Raphe. See *Median raphe.*

Red blood cell (corpuscle, erythrocyte). A non-nucleated biconcave cell bearing hemoglobin and responsible for transport of oxygen to tissues via the circulatory system.

Reduced enamel epithelium. The several layers of the epithelial enamel organ compacted and remaining on the surface of enamel after enamel formation is complete.

Remodeling. Alteration of the structure by reconstruction. The continuous process of turnover of bone carried out by osteoblasts and osteoclasts.

Reparative dentin (tertiary dentin). Deposition of new dentin in response to disease or pulpal trauma. A defensive reaction whereby hard tissue formation walls off the pulp from the site of injury.

RER. See *Rough endoplasmic reticulum (RER).*

Reticulum. Smooth surface endoplasmic reticulum, composed of flat double membrane sheets of protoplasmic reticulum. No ribosomes on its outer surface.

Retzius' striae. Lines reflecting successive incremental deposition of mineralized enamel.

Reversal lines. Lines separating layers of bone or cementum deposited in a resorption site distinguishing it from the scalloped outline of Howship's lacunae.

Ribosomes. Particles that translate genetic codes for proteins and activate mechanisms for their production.

RNA (ribonucleic acid). Carries information to sites of actual protein synthesis located in the cell cytoplasm.

Root canal. Extension of the pulp from the coronal zone to the root apex. See also *Accessory root canal.*

Root resorption. Dissolution of the root of a tooth by action of osteoclasts. This may occur anywhere along the surface of the tooth root in response to caries or trauma or during the loss of a primary tooth.

Root sheath cells (Hertwig's sheath). Merged outer and inner epithelial layers of the enamel organ, extending beyond the region of the crown to invest the developing root.

Root trunk. The part of the tooth immediately below the crown neck before division into the roots, covered by cementum and fixed in the alveolus.

Rough endoplasmic reticulum (RER) (granular). The ribosomes attached to the endoplasmic reticulum that function in synthesis of secretory protein.

Ruffled border. An area enfolding the plasma membrane of the osteoclast that borders the resorptive zone.

Saliva. Clear, slightly alkaline, somewhat viscid mixture of secretions of the salivary glands and gingival fluid exudate. It moistens the mucous membranes and food, facilitating speech and mastication. Consists of water and 0.58 percent solids.

Salivary calculi. Calcium phosphate concentrations (salivary stones or sialolithiasis) found within a salivary gland or duct, most commonly in the main excretory duct of the submandibular gland (Wharton's duct).

Salivary corpuscle. One of the leukocytes or lymphocytes found in saliva.

Salivary gland. Exocrine glands whose secretions flow into the oral cavity.

Schwann cell. Cell forming the myelin sheath of nerves and seen in association with all nerves of the pulp.

Sclerotic (transparent) dentin. Dentin in which the tubules are occluded with mineral. Occurs mostly in elderly people, especially in the roots of teeth.

Sclerotomes. Part of the somite consisting of mesenchymal tissue that develops into vertebrae and ribs.

Secondary dentin. Circumpulpal deposition of dentin formed after tooth eruption.

Secondary palate. The palate proper formed by fusion of the lateral palatine processes of the maxilla.

Serous. Relating to, containing, or producing a serum substance with a watery consistency.

Serous demilunes. Half-moon or crescent-shaped serous cells associated with the terminal external surface or mucous alveoli.

Serous glands of tongue (von Ebner's). Serous glands opening into the bottom of the trough surrounding the circumvallate papillae and functioning in a cleansing

Serumal calculus. Subgingival calculus so termed because it results in part from exudation of serum.

Sharpey's fibers. See *Perforating fibers (Sharpey's fibers).*

Sialography. Diagnostic x-ray technique for visualizing salivary gland ducts by injection of a radiopaque substance into the main excretory duct.

Smooth muscle cells. Cells whose contractility is under control of the autonomic nervous system.

Soft palate. Posterior muscular portion of the palate, forming an incomplete septum between the nasopharynx and the oral cavity.

Somites. Paired blocklike masses of mesoderm arranged segmentally along the neural tube in the embryo and forming the dermis, vertebral column, and musculature.

Specialized mucosa. Mucosa found on the dorsum of the tongue that consists of four types of papillae: filiform, fungiform, circumvallate, and foliate.

Spindles. The termination of dentinal tubules in inner enamel.

Squamous. Relating to the flat squama, as of the temporal bone.

Squamous epithelium. Composed of a single layer of flat scalelike cells, as in the lining of the pulmonary alveoli, or stratified as in oral epithelium.

Stellate reticulum. A network of star-shaped cells in the center of the enamel organ between the outer and inner enamel epithelia.

Stensen's duct. The epithelium-lined duct that drains the parotid gland.

Stomodeum. The future oral cavity of the embryo; an invagination lined by surface ectoderm.

Stratified epithelium. A type of epithelium composed of a series of layers. The cells of each may vary in size and shape, as seen in skin and some mucous membranes.

Stratum intermedium. Epithelial cell layer of the enamel organ that lies external and adjacent to the inner enamel epithelium and attached to it by desmosomes. Stratum intermedium also refers to the intermediate layer of nonkeratinizing epithelia.

Striae of Retzius. See *Retzius' striae.*

Striated duct. An intralobular salivary secretory gland duct involved in ionic transport, located between the intercalated and interlobular ducts, and named for the basal striations produced by the enfoldings of the basal membrane within the cells.

Stroma. Supporting framework of a gland, such as the capsule and trabeculae, rather than the functional parenchyma.

Sublingual. Refers to the area beneath the anterior lower jaw.

Sublingual gland. The smallest of the three pairs of major salivary glands. A pure mucous gland located in the anterior floor of the mouth.

Submandibular. Refers to the area beneath the angle of the mandible.

Submandibular gland. One of the three paired major salivary glands that contributes 65 percent of saliva. These bilateral glands are a mixed seromucous type.

Submucosa. Layer of tissues that lies beneath the lamina propria underlying the mucous membrane of the lip, cheek, palate, and floor of the mouth.

Successional lamina. That portion of the dental lamina lingual to the developing deciduous teeth. It gives rise to the enamel organs of permanent teeth.

Supporting bone. Bone tissue functionally related to supporting the roots of the teeth. It surrounds, protects, and supports the tooth roots through the alveolar bone proper.

Sympathetic nervous system. The thoracolumbar part of the autonomic nervous system. Preganglionic fibers arise from cell bodies in the thoracic and first three lumbar segments of the spinal cord. Postganglionic fibers are distributed to the heart, smooth muscle, and glands of the entire body.

Synapse. The region of the junction between two nerve cells where an impulse passes between the axon of one cell and the dendrite of another cell.

Synchondrosis. A type of cartilaginous joint that usually is temporary.

Syndesmosis. A type of fibrous joint in which opposing surfaces are united by fibrous connective tissue, as in the union between most facial bones.

Synovial membranes. Membranes that line joint cavities and secrete a small amount of clear, transparent alkaline fluid in the articular spaces. Synovial fluid acts as a lubricant and nutrient for the avascular tissue covering, that is, the condyle and articular tubercle of the temporomandibular joint; also called synovial fluid.

T cells. Cells produced by the thymus that destroy invading microbes and are therefore important to the body's immune system.

Taste bud. Receptor of taste on the tongue and in the oropharynx. One of several goblet-shaped cells oriented at right angles to the surface by the epithelium. They consist of supporting and gustatory cells.

Temporomandibular joint. Joint formed between the condyle of the mandible and the mandibular fossa (concavity of the temporal bone).

Temporomandibular ligaments. Four ligaments: the sphenomandibular, on the medial surface; the stylomandibular, on the posterior surface; the temporomandibular, on the lateral surface; and the capsular, surrounding the joint.

Teratogen. Agent or factor that produces physical defects in the developing embryo.

Terminal bar apparatus. Localized condensations of cytoplasmic substance associated with the cell membrane of the apical area of the functional ameloblast.

Tertiary dentin. See *Reparative dentin (tertiary dentin).*

TMJ. See *Temporomandibular joint.*

Tomes' granular layer. This layer of dentin is found only in the tooth root. It is adjacent to the peripheral zone of hyalinized root dentin as a thin, hypomineralized layer.

Tomes' process. Specialized apical zone of the ameloblasts. Tomes' process is conical and interdigitates with the forming enamel rods.

Tonofibrils. Systems of fibers found in the cytoplasm of epithelial cells, which function with the desmosomal plaque to hold adjacent cells together.

Tooth crypt. Space filled by the dental follicle and developing tooth within the alveolar process.

Tooth eruption. Process by which teeth emerge into the oral cavity; a stage coordinated with root growth and maturation of tissues surrounding the tooth.

Traction bands of the palate. Bundles of collagen fibers that firmly attach the oral mucosa to the underlying bone of the hard palate.

Transduction theory. Proposes that odontoblasts are sensory receptors for pain stimuli that are transmitted through the dentin.

Transparent dentin. See *Sclerotic dentin.*

Tuft. See *Enamel tuft.*

Vasculature. Refers to the blood vessels and circulating blood system.

Vermilion border. The exposed red portion of the lips. This color is due to a thin epithelium, with the presence of eleidin in the cells and the superficial position of the blood vessels.

Vestibular lamina. Lip furrow band located labial and buccal to the dental lamina; forms the oral vestibule between the alveolar portions of the jaws and the lips and cheeks.

Viscerocranial. Refers to those parts of the facial cranial skeleton originating from the branchial arch.

Volkmann's canals. These "perforating canals" enter the bone at right or oblique angles and establish a continuous system that contains the nerves and blood vessels of bone.

Vomer. Flat, unpaired bone located in the midline of the face, shaped like a trapezoid, and forming the inferior and posterior portions of the nasal septum. It articulates with the sphenoid, ethmoid, two maxillary, and two palatine bones.

Von Ebner's lines. See *Imbrication lines.*

Waldeyer's ring. A ring of tonsillary tissue surrounding the oropharynx. It is composed of palatine tonsils located laterally—the lingual in the floor of the mouth and the pharyngeal in the posterior area of the pharynx.

Weil's basal layer. See *Cell-free zone.*

Wharton's duct. The duct that drains the submandibular gland.

Zygoma. The process of the temporal bone that connects with the zygomatic bone.

Zygote. The fertilized cell produced by the union of two gametes.

Zymogen. An inactive precursor that is activated to an enzyme. Granules in serous cells of enzyme-secreting glands, such as the salivary glands and the pancreas.

Index